SCOTT GILLET,

TRUE BUD

UNDERSTANDING TOXIC MARIJUANA SYNDROME

BIRD

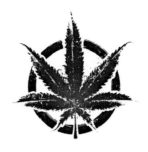

ACKNOWLEDGEMENTS

The Briarcliff Institute for Recovery and Development (BIRD) is a small outpatient institute with a small staff that works as a team on most cases. Our resources for a project this large were limited and if not for the help of Dr. Wilson from ARL, Ian Jenkins and Dr. Morris from Systemic Formulas, and Kate Wells and Dr. Ross from Labrix we would have never been able to move forward. In addition, the financial and emotional support of my father was incredible! I want to note that at the time I was conducting the research and writing this book my mother was progressing into the later stages of Alzheimer's disease. I was extremely grateful for my father's support when he was going through the most difficult time in his life. I am truly touched by his belief in the TMS project and in the Briarcliff Institute. I would also like to thank Jenna Gillet for assistance in getting the tests out to the necessary people and Dr. Tricia Clauser for assisting the institute in so many ways throughout the years including helping launch this book.

Finally, I would be remise not to mention the huge support of our kids. These young clients new something was not right in their brains and bodies due to heavy, chronic use of weed as well as light recreational use of dabs and wax. Their candidness and bravery are to be commended. They even let me cut their hair!!! The hair had to be cut in a specific way in order to collect reliable samples for the hair testing. I think they can all attest to the fact that I am NOT a hairdresser! I would like to thank my three children; Jenna, Sarah, and Sam for coming up with a great title for this book!

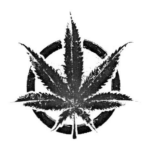

TABLE OF CONTENTS

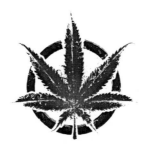

Introduction

Throughout my experience working with young people over the years I began to see a real pattern in the chronic marijuana users. I have come to firmly believe chronic weed use is a kind of trauma to the mind, body, family system, and spirit of these young people. The levels of toxicity from various sources which will be revealed in this book is leading to major impacts on brain chemistry. What is thought of as a benign substance by many young people as well as their parents, when used chronically (multiple times daily) is in fact not benign at all. Trauma has a major impact on one's life and the systems the individual interacts in. Young people have very little level of awareness of the harmful effects weed and dabs have when used chronically. This book will illustrate how and why we are making these statements. Research was conducted and testing revealed so many aspects contradicting the popular belief that weed is a benign substance. The brain is a fragile place and was never meant to consume a substance like dabs, K2, spice, or chemicals in metal bongs. Young people including their cognitive functioning and family system is being altered by chronic marijuana use. They often refer to themselves as stoners and laugh.

Information in this book revealing the impact and truth of what is unfolding in chronic users indicates that being a stoner may not be a laughing matter at all. This is not to discount some of the beneficial uses of marijuana when grown organically and monitored responsibly. Clearly, medical marijuana has a place in our society as you will see when you read about the Israelis and all they have done to regulate the medical marijuana industry. This book goes into many issues surrounding abusive bud use as well as the positive effects of marijuana.

It is my belief that chronic weed use, with so many unknowns, is a trauma to the young person's brain, body, and spirit. The system was never meant to I ingest these high levels of toxins that do not get removed and I feel it is traumatizing young people leading to the development of TMS. My concern is that we may be losing a generation of young people who call themselves stoners who are severely addicted to weed. This book will not argue the merits of whether marijuana is addictive or not and will not look at the recreational user. It is the chronic, addicted weed users that we are concerned about. We are also concerned that medical marijuana, which was meant to alleviate suffering and is useful for that, has at times found to be toxic. My true passion lies with helping the younger generations live a full life accomplishing all of their hopes and dreams. I hope this book sheds some light on what I believe to be a very serious detriment to our youth.

TMS= Toxic Marijuana Syndome

chronic =

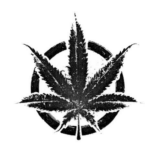

PROCEDURE

A small group of the BIRD clients, between the ages of 17-25, agreed to allow me to test them for TMS. I will refer to them as the BIRD six. All of them were chronic weed users who blazed more than once daily. All six participants had used Dabs, the highly concentrated form of bud that is often used by butane-cooper tanks. They had also used very similar strains of weed. Participants were asked to complete a survey developed by one of our therapists, Jeff Munk, LCSW to identify TMS. I felt that all of the participants in this study were authentic and honest in disclosure.

In addition to the survey there were three tests administered to each participant:

1. The tissue mineral test analysis by Analytical research labs, Inc. with assistance of Dr. Wilson and Kathleen Korda, HHP - hair test
2. The Kryptopyrrole disorder test by Direct Health Care Access, Inc. - urine test
3. The Neurotransmitter repot test by Labrix labs with the assistance of Kate Wells and Dr. Ross

An explanation of the process including the use and purpose of the above tests was provided to all participants and their parents (if under 18 years of age). Written consent was obtained from all participants. BIRD paid for all testing of these young people. Systemic Formulas, a great Nutrient company, was extremely helpful and also provided the treatment protocols for dealing with what these tests revealed. I found the labs and staff from all very helpful. Funding for testing was provided by my father, Harold Gillet, who believes in the work BIRD is doing around TMS. Labrix was very helpful and did not even charge us for the first round of tests which I am grateful for.

During the course of putting this book together we started our own research on Bud and the impact on the brain. This research is ongoing. Our findings are here in the book in the chapter entitled, Testing the BIRD Six. Results of testing revealed high levels of toxins such as copper, mercury, aluminum, manganese, and phosphorus. Low zinc levels were also revealed. Two out of the six participant placed high in the disorder known as Kryptopyrrole. I did find that these test results were helpful in creating abstinence in several of our young people. Five out of the six participants had major nutrient deficiency. These tests were enough to convince me that the TMS project and testing was going to be a useful tool for treatment of chronic weed users. Although not meant to scare the kids, the results did shake them up and motivate them towards abstinence. Perhaps testing is a tool that can help other chronic weed users in the future.

Future research should consider incorporating blood testing into the process. Ideally, I would have liked to incorporate blood testing into this project, but the blood work would demand a long drive to another state and our participants were just not willing to go there.

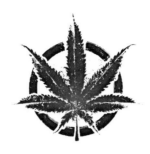

Understanding
the Brain Simply

Let's take a look at the brain and how it works in a simple, non-complicated way. It's important for you to know what's happening up there. We will begin by looking at the major players in brain functions:

The Prefrontal Lobe: This is where evaluation takes place. It is the area of the brain responsible for reasoning and receiving information from outside stimuli and also from other parts of the brain. It is a major player in regulating and helping with emotions, control, and choices.

Amygdala: Also known as the coordination center. It has two almond shaped groups of neuron's that also are major players. Each section has its own functions. The right one is located in the temporal mode. It takes in fear situations, threats or events like a trauma. Its location allows it to receive and send information to other parts of the brain and is often included as part of the limbic system. The right almond shaped part helps to coordinate emotional and psychological responses. This part of the Amygdala is where you have your fight or flight response as well as something referred to as the frozen response. Thus, when hit with a stressful event or an accident, it will help you with one of the three; fight, flight, or freeze. All-important survival mechanisms are housed here. Some new research indicates that the amygdala takes a picture of major events and sends it to be stored in another part of the brain. This is to protect an individual during times of stress when they may not want to remember a specific picture, right then and there, but may want to access it at a later time

The Hippocampus: This part of the limbic system is responsible for learning and storing information. It also assists with retrieval of an event. It will assist the Amygdala in memory and emotion expression and helps to connect things up to the other parts of the brain.

The Thalamus: Receives and sends sensory information and helps with modulation by other brain centers.

The Cingulate Gyrus: Related to orientating the brain to an incoming stimulus or threat and stands at attention at all times.

The Hypothalamus: Involved with the release of stress hormones, like cortisol and adrenaline. When it receives incoming information of a major event, like that you just had a car accident, those chemicals will be given the green light to become released and assist you in that event. During this time the amygdala is photographing the event and picking what works best; fight, flight, or freeze.

*Released hormones need to be replenished when depleted.

The Prefrontal Cortex: Also plays a role in reasoning and it serves as an inhibitor of responses arising from the limbic system. It evaluates threats and does some reasoning regarding how to handle certain situations. The prefrontal cortex is always at work, but is deeply affected by things like low blood sugar, drinking, smoking marijuana, and using other drugs. Its job as inhibitor slacks off when under the influence!!

Those are the major players for our purpose here. Let's move on to the brain and memory:

We have two major types of memory. The first is the Declarative Memory which relies on the Hippocampus for its information and factual experience. The second is the Procedural Memory which deals with our earlier memories and not the here and now. Declarative deals with memory around the here and now. The Procedural Memory incorporates feelings from getting sensory input on emotional events coming from those pictures in the amygdala. The brain needs Glutamate from its receptor sites for memory to work right.

The other important work of the brain takes place in the receptor sites. The major neurotransmitters include GABA, Dopamine, Endorphins, Serotonin, and Acetylcholine. There are others neurotransmitters found in the brain, however these have a lot to do with how we feel. The levels of these sites are important to being a healthy person and overall mental stability. Some people are born with lower levels at their receptor sites while others have high levels. Some may deplete the site thru things like addiction. Some can improve the firing of these sites thru amino acids, yoga, exercise, sex, rock climbing, swimming, and being in love. Even having a dog. A study showed that having a dog raises a chemical we make called oxytocin. Oxytocin is a feel good chemical. I personally can attest to its impact as I recently adopted a dog, Shanti. Since he has entered my life my oxytocin levels have gone up.

The following are the characteristics of the neurotransmitter sites. There are 100 neurotransmitter sites, but I will define the main ones here:

Dopamine - alertness, motivation, and energy to do things in life. Creates movement and is affected by chronic weed use.

Serotonin - helps with sensory input. Provides us with a sense. Derived from Tryptophan and provides a feeling of well-being. Allows us to feel safe. When lowered it causes depression. All of the new SSRIs are geared towards raising this site. Effected by chronic weed use.

Endorphin - This is where the opiate site is. It helps regulate how we deal with pain in life. When in crisis it releases endorphins to help with the oncoming crisis or pain event. There are many ways to raise this site including two of the most basics, sex and exercise.

Gaba - Known as the calming neurotransmitter. It helps regulate stress. It calms and relaxes us. Weed use will raise Gaba, but chronic weed use will deplete it.

Norepinephrine - Regulates mood and anxiety, retrieval of information is essential to inhibit the outflow from the pre frontal cortex to the amygdala. Shifts the behavior to the amygdala. Norepinephrine and dopamine are catecholamines. It is also a stress hormone. Norepinephrine was found to be low in our weed users.

Trauma can impact receptor sites as it impacts the amygdala. A series of ongoing traumas can deplete serotonin. Having just one trauma can deplete anyone of the neurotransmitters. Post-traumatic stress disorder (PTSD) also will impact the site due to it being a brain event, even if the incident was physical. It is important to heal trauma on a brain chemistry level. The topic of trauma and bud use will be covered more extensively in the chapter Trauma Buds.

If you would like to know more about ways to improve your brain I recommend the work of Dr.'s Amen, Perlmutter, Hyla Cass, and Ruden who have written great books that will impact you in a positive way. In Dr. Perlmutter's book he states that our environment, stress, and chemicals change and influence the brain and DNA structure. He states that the brain can be repaired and that we even have the ability to grow new brain cells thru lifestyle changes, nutrients, food. Swami Satchidanada, a world renowned Yoga master, often would say, "Change your life and you will change everything in your cell structure and you're firing in your brain." The Swami was an incredible example of the ability to create change in thousands of people by his teachings and presence.

Epigenetics can impact the brain and the DNA. What we do today impacts future generations in our family systems. All of the doctors mentioned, in addition to others I have studied with, feel that certain key nutrients are essential in today's world. They all feel everyone belongs on Omega 3DHA, for example. There are also other yoga practices that may help, but I would only use them with a mentor or teacher who has been thru this dealing with trauma with others.

Jnana Yoga is the practice of "Who Am I." Am I this event that I had little control over? Am I this body and brain that may have been impacted by the event? This practice was made by Ramana Maharshi, a great saint in India who taught this to all his students. He helped them develop a witness state where they could witness the trauma, the mind and the body's reactions, without engaging in the story or charges that the event creates. Thru deep meditation, one would reach a clear, calm and somewhat serene space and from that space, all could be witnessed without emotion. The brain could also be taught to become calm and accepting around the event, once the charge was gone. Again, this is for long time students of yoga with a skillful teacher and not meant to do on your own. Somatic healing, using deep breath work, a trained therapist relaxes your body and helps you reach a semi trance like state where deep breathing stays throughout the processes. Images may come up and sensations from the body may come up surrounding events from the trauma. One needs to be in a place and try to be willing to let go. As they come up, the triggers are dealt with in a loving way, accepted, and felt in a gentle way. Time takes its time. No rush and sessions will build to a place of trust and release over time. The therapist will often write down things if they interact with the client as they may in some sessions. It is thought that the amygdala will release during somatic sessions.

Observation has taught me that when it comes to trauma each brain and emotional person is different. It is a process to learn and see what works best for each individual. Talking about the event too soon after the event at times will not work. It is almost like the brain is on lock down and needs to protect itself and survive. The person may just need more time before they begin the therapy and healing process. Pushing one into treatment too fast, when they are not ready is not a good thing based on how the brain works. It is also important to understand that all traumas are linked in the brain and emotional body. They are not separate. It is almost if joined by a string and dealing with one event will often unleash other buried events that are stored in the amygdala. A person can begin to speak or work around one recent event and suddenly be back in something long forgotten from childhood that is coming up for the first time just now. One must be very gentle with this, it is totally out of the person's control.

Finally, what is our attitude? How do we deal with challenges? What are our connections in life, our spirituality, our commitment to service and helping those in need? There is no limit to the amount of love you can feel. That choice is up to you. Love changes everything!!!

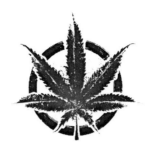

THE TEEN BRAIN

There has been a lot of recent work on the teen brain. We now have the use of MRIs, PET scans, and super scans that can create images of the brain. Adolescence is a time of huge brain growth and changes when a multitude of wiring and complex events occur. Synaptic pruning, deployment of the prefrontal cortex, is one major event. Also occurring at this time are developments in impulse control, decision making, thought processing, planning, memory, and the balancing of hormones and emotions that are surging and soaring. The major growth period of the brain is between the ages 13 and 26 years old. This is also the age at which the majority of young people begin to experiment with marijuana and other substances.

The prefrontal cortex goes thru a huge growth spurt at which point thinking, rather than acting on things, becomes part of its job. By the age of 17, 80% of the brain is almost fully developed. Cells are activated as children engage in life. The major tasks of young people and how they will do these tasks is unfolding. Mood, attention, and the importance of impulse control based on mood and hormones are part of this task. Problem solving is being learned and built during these years. It is a very vulnerable time for young people due to fluctuation of hormone levels and emerging sexuality. Synaptic events are common and the brain is just beginning to connect myelination in the frontal lobe. Judgment around choices in life develop during this time.

Research has shown that girls develop two years ahead of boys. All of this growth will continue until approximately 26 years of age. How trauma is going to be dealt with also develops in the part of the brain known as the Amygdala as the fight, flight, or freeze instincts emerge. Addiction is a learned response developing during this time as the brain is learning an incredible amount. Some of these young brains are already susceptible to addiction through genetic coding and DNA factors and Epigenetics. The teen brain is vulnerable to any substances used during this time, because substance use (even recreational) will leave an imprint.

Marijuana has a huge impact on the brain. The brain has cannabis receptor sites and marijuana use will impact those sites. Memory is hugely affected at a time when the brain is trying to learn as much as it can. The brain responds to substances in the reward center. Images have shown how areas of the brain light up in the reward center when a substance is introduced. Risk taking is a major task children have to learn to work thru adolescents. The ability to acknowledge choices and make decisions is another important factor as information gets moved to the prefrontal cortex. Marijuana will impair this ability having a major impact on the prefrontal cortex.

It is also important to note that the Amygdala is hugely impacted by marijuana. As noted previously, the Amygdala is an incredibly important part of the brain responsible for handling trauma and fight or flight. It is also responsible for releasing major chemicals such as cortisol, epinephrine, and other hormones which will not be able to perform their natural process if a child is high on marijuana.

Our culture is putting more and more pressure on the young brain. My feeling is that it can often not keep up. As it gets stressed, chemicals get released, and marijuana serves a purpose in calming the processes down. It is important not to judge this, but to educate children about their own brain functioning and help them learn if they are at risk for marijuana abuse. Over 22 years, Dr. Amen conducted 83,000 brain scans. He has the largest amount of data collected on behavior and how drugs impact the brain. Scans show that children's brains respond differently to things and many of his treatment plans reflect what these scans show. I highly recommend you read and look at his work. My feeling used to be based on a family systems model in treating children, but over the years I have taken the time to learn how their brains and thinking works and how epigenetics, trauma, and multi-generationally family DNA coding impacts things as well.

We are seeing more and more senseless acts of mass violence committed by young people, more suicide and more addiction than ever before. It is difficult to come up with a reason why a child would go into a school and kill his classmates, but we are deeply troubled by the alarming rate of young people doing this. Bad and evil behavior can be associated with major brain chemistry events and we need to start to look at this more closely. There is no excuse for such senseless violence, but brain scans would reveal a lot and brain testing even more. Changes in brain chemistry is attainable. Out of all the drugs around, marijuana leaves a huge trail. Most drugs are out of the brain quickly, but not marijuana. It is also important to consider what is in the marijuana. Was it laced? Was it the highly potent dabs at 80% THC? Was it sprayed with pesticides meant for lawns and trees and not fit for any human consumption?

The frontal lobe of the brain is not fully connected to its other parts until approximately age 25. With addiction being a learned behavior the brain can easily trick itself into believing that marijuana is good for it. I have seen it where marijuana helps children with ADHD in early use manage anxiety, lower social inhibitions, and deal with those isolating feelings children go thru. Studies have shown that children who smoke marijuana will have cognitive impairment days later after use, due to the trail marijuana leaves. Studies have also shown that marijuana impacts the teen brain differently than the formed adult brain.

Another part of the brain, the hippocampus, is still being formed in the young brain. This part of the brain has a huge area of the CB1 cannabinoid receptor sites. The hippocampus is responsible for learning and memory. Studies have shown that hippocampal neuronal assemblies, when linked to cannabinoid input, induced memory impairment and morphological changes from any type of ongoing marijuana use. This also included major gene expression and hippocampal protein expression.

An expert in young brain development at the National Institute of Mental Health, Dr. Jay Giedd, studied 145 MRI brain scans of children. He observed a large amount of synaptic pruning. The prefrontal cortex serves as the CEO of the brain. Control, planning, executive functioning, organizational planning, and some mood regulation occur here. Dr. Giedd hypothesized that the growth in gray matter followed by the pruning of connections is a most important stage of brain development at a point which the choices teens make can affect them for the rest of their lives. He calls it the "Use it or Lose it" factor. Heavy marijuana use during this time will impair this processes and if the marijuana is laced or has high levels of toxins from pesticides, the functioning can be hugely impacted. The idea that a brain can be polluted before it is even given chance to grow and become whatever it was meant to be is tragic.

There is also major growth in the corpus callosum throughout adolescents. The corpus callosum is the part of the brain involved in information relating and transferring important information between the hemispheres. The cerebellum is susceptible to marijuana use which can impact the information being transferred. Teen brain studies show information also moves from the back of the brain to the prefrontal cortex which is in the frontal part of the brain. Connections are trimmed down by synaptic pruning, then the protective coating, called myelin coats, assist the synapses. Marijuana can impact the connection process by attaching to fat soluble cells and the myelin sheath and remaining in the brain for long periods of time after use.

The reward center in the teen's brain is in the nucleus acumens and is thought to be fully developed by the time a child reaches adolescents. At times we can have a very strong reward center and an underdeveloped prefrontal cortex. When a reward is too powerful it is not unusual for the prefrontal cortex to have difficulty maintaining impulse control. Things like food, sex, drugs, money, and of course rock and roll or rap can easily override the prefrontal cortex. This is the beginning of addiction on a brain chemistry level.

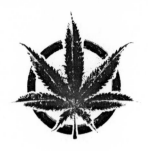

TRAUMA BUDS

It is inevitable that young people will experience a trauma while going from adolescence into adulthood. Trauma experienced by an adolescent is processed differently than that of an adult. Many Trauma survivors result to abusing substance in order to cope with the pain. The young brain is in motion, evolving and always changing. Adolescents is a pivotal time for brain development and Trauma can gravely impact this growth. A few traumas an adolescent may experience include; explosive divorces, domestic violence, physical and sexual, partner abuse, auto accidents, sports injuries, loss of friends or family from drug use or suicide. As time in treatment goes by and trust is developed, these traumas are uncovered.

We know that trauma is a brain event along with body, feelings, emotions and the spirit.

As a clinician who works with young substance abusers, I am often faced with the reality of the trauma survivor, who prior to the event never smoked marijuana, after the event becomes highly addicted using marijuana as their own survival mechanism. It becomes a vicious cycle where young people resort to marijuana use to facilitate the coping process but it in turn inhibits their ability to process the trauma and move on from it. They instead become detached from themselves rather than connecting to their inner pain. The marijuana does not make the memory and pain of the trauma go away it just numbs the pain for the time being, allowing it to fester. For those who experience continuous trauma, they have explained to me a certain disconnect from the event, almost as if it were not real. Kind of like a film running without catching the emotionally content. The young people who have recalled these events to me say that their body was present during the trauma but their mind was not 100% present. That the weed protected them from the full force of trauma and for them that was a good thing. We know that trauma can deplete the brain, that it effects receptor cite activity and stress hormones like cortisol. With chronic marijuana users trauma is hitting an already depleted brain.

The chapter "Understanding the Brain Simply" maps out the functions and tasks of specific parts of the brain. A huge player in any trauma event is the part of the brain called the amygdala. Our fight, flight or frozen state exists in the amygdala. I see and hear very little fight, not much fight, but a lot of frozen. A frozen state where the young person is unable to do anything with the stimuli coming in. I have seen kids come in with the news of a close friend's death and be completely frozen. They will describe a feeling of numbness and wonder how they can feel so little at a time of such sadness. I recall a night where a local youth had taken his own life. The peers and friends wanted a place to come and process. As it was, some of the kids attending our groups were close friends and the institute became the spot to come and talk in a group forum, with little structure, rules, guidelines or heavy staff involvement. Most of the group was frozen solid. Most were high and for many there was a level of awareness that they were really not feeling, not too emotionally charged. Early grief will often look like this, particularly in young people. However, what I was seeing and hearing that night was those stoned were unable to participate fully in the event because THC was jamming something up in their heads impacting their emotions. It was a violent sudden death. A real shock for them and the community. It was also a very important moment in their young lives for deeper learning and beginning to understand their feelings and how they worked.

It may help an individual to not feel, but that is tragic in itself. To not be able to feel and for the brain not to go through the normal process when it experiences big hit is particularly sad for a therapist to behold. Such a missed moment. To add insult to injury, the young people know this and judge themselves for being so wasted during major moments. During that night those kids came and shared the experience of death with us. I was not surprised to find kids coming and going and moving around a lot, thawing as words were spoken that perhaps could help them get unstuck.

So much has happened in trauma work. So many new and exciting treatments on all levels including brain, body, spirit, and emotions. We know have access to techniques such as brain remapping, EMDR, Emotional Freedom Techniques (EFT), working with Metadata, nuerofeedback, timelines, 12 step models for trauma survivors, holistic approaches such as yoga and meditation. There are inpatient treatment centers all across the US that just work with trauma victims. There are doctors and Nutrient Therapists treating brain depletion with aminos and nutrients in the diet. There are so many spiritual types of support. There is such a huge reservoir to draw upon. However, time is a big factor in processing trauma and time is distorted with weed use. Our belief is simple, the substance weed has to stop. Brain chemistry needs to be repaired and toxicity removed, feelings restored, emotions regulated, and a total shift in body and spirit. Within each individual there is the ability to heal and become restored.

Once restored, we can take a look at that picture the amygdala took and saved, initiate the trauma work, and a new life will begin to form.

Based on years of working with chronic and recreational young bud users of every kind, it is my strong belief that many young people are developing something that I call Toxic Marijuana Syndrome (TMS). It is my belief that chronic marijuana use is a trauma to the young person's brain, body, and spirit. The chemicals in pesticides as well as the paraphernalia used to smoke marijuana are negatively impacting the brain chemistry of our young people. It is a difficult thing to see so many young people having so many problems as a result of marijuana use. The traumatizing impact on our youth is leading to the development of TMS which will be illustrated in the following chapter on the TMS sheet. For those of you who may not be familiar with trauma and how it manifests itself I have provided a little information on how the disorder is experienced as well as treated.

Experiencing Post-Traumatic Stress Disorder

PTSD - The following are some of the challenges the traumatized person will have to deal with:

1. Re-experiencing the trauma - This is always connected to any other traumas they might have had at any time in the life cycle.
2. Emotional Numbing - This shutting down of emotions operate like a switch when the fight, flight or frozen states are triggered by anything associated with the traumas. This is like a switch that shuts off the currents of emotions, a form of protection, due to too much stimulus coming in. The person often has little control of this and enters a frozen state. Defrosting must come from a skillful therapist who understands and works with trauma, timing is a huge factor.

19

3. Avoidance - The person will create movement in their life to not trigger the wound. They will stay away from people, places, and things. They will not drive down certain roads and will avoid any events even remotely connected to the trauma. Some will move and relocate, while some will be afraid of emotional intimacy for fear of recreating any new kind of wounding.

4. Denial - A person is capable of putting the trauma event away somewhere inside, like a compartment and they can easily train themselves, thru avoidance, to believe that event never occurred. The mind and brain are so powerful, that a hijacking can take the person over. Denying any trauma prevents hijacking and gives the illusion of safety to them. It is very much like the frozen state, but it is not bad or wrong, just a form of survival protection. We as clinicians must learn to be both patient and compassionate and let time and the work do their thing. Everything must come from a loving place, the person is fragile.

5. Hypersensitivity and an increased sense of arousal - As the person's awareness returns after an event they can be different in their levels of sensitivity. They have little control over this, it is a brain chemistry event. Their organism is on alert for danger now and this heightened state is their new survival mechanism that they feel they must trust it. It can be feelings, kinetic, sounds, sights, and things that can't be explained or understood, except by the traumatized person. They are going to be personalizing things more and this may be very different than how they were before the event. It is possible they may not be able to walk thru Times Square or be on a train. Sensory overload just kicks in for no real reason. This can be one of the most challenging aspects of PTSD due to the lack of

understanding or compassion of their friends, coworkers, and family members. They may be trying too hard to get the person back into the flow of life, and they feel they are being kind and supportive, but they are not. Hypersensitivity can become very painful for the person and this is a big reason why so many PTSD people move into substance abuse and use, to create a layer between themselves and the outside world. Their use is a form of filtering and protection from the raw state of feeling and seeing and sensing everything around them. This is a human phenomenon and does not exist in animals. Although, I am not sure if that applies to dogs. The dog I have, Shanti is very smart and sensitive due to several near death experiences, beyond our control. At times he does seem triggered by some things and will not move and remains in his frozen state and often moves towards me for comfort and reassurance in a triggered moment. While watching the dog whisperer, Cesar Millan, I was amazed at how skillful he was with traumatized dogs and by how much he understood their inner world and the shift that needed to take place for change and resolution. He spoke a lot about what the dog's brain was doing in this moment as he worked his magic

6. Losing problem solving skills - Due to mental confusion, fear, not trusting themselves or others, many people lose the simple task of problem solving. Things seem bigger and challenging on many levels. They may go to friends and family with what looks like a very easy problem to solve, but the brain has had a brain event and is not functioning at its peak level and needs time and some brain repair work to restore it to its natural state. Some brains get there, some don't. So many chemicals are released in areas of the brain, that what was once simple is

now hard due to the loss of some of those chemicals. Engaging a coach for a while would assist them as they move towards healing their process

7. A new level of brain fog and some mental confusion - Again the brain has been impacted during the event or events and like a computer that has a virus or needs more memory, the brain cannot keep up with all the incoming information and stimulus. At times certain key nutrients can help and support getting the brain back to its proper functioning level. I am not a big fan of medications for trauma, although at times there is no choice. The reason why is that the resetting works better when it is a natural event and meds tend to dull, limit, and only move the feelings and thinking about what happened to the person to a part of the brain and body that we need access to for healing. Nutrients and key Amino acids in higher doses, on the other hand, just mimic the brains natural ability to restore. Remember, there is a loss of key chemicals that support brain function and focus needs to be on that part of the healing also. I have never seen a case of someone traumatized who does not have brain fog, even if they're in denial or avoidance.

8. Nightmares, parasomnia, insomnia, flashbacks, intrusive thoughts, nighttime waking and eating or medicating, even sleepwalking - When our systems are shut down at night and we are in the REM sleep state, the subconscious and unconscious parts of our minds and brain come into play and rise up. This again is not a bad thing, although it is very challenging for the person going thru it and we need to be very sensitive to it. We can also use it to promote healing. It is almost like they are re-experiencing the original trauma. I was a sleepwalker and I love to talk to other sleepwalkers, because it has helped me learn

much more about what sleepwalking is. Often, my parents or sister would have to go up to the roof of the apartment building we lived in and wake me up before I fell off the roof. I once woke up in a neighbor's bathtub, and when woken, I truly thought I was in my bed. The craziest walk I ever had was from our place to the downtown area, where the police picked me up and were not sure what to do with me or who I belonged to, because I was only seven and in my PJs and was not carrying any ID. Sleep walking is not a crime, so it was all good and they got me home, but told my parents that if it happened again, I would have to wear some tags. Like dog tags!!! At times, when woken by a flashback, it is better to try and feel, process and maybe call a friend if they are okay with a call in the middle of the night hoping they know the deal and are okay with that. Those in 12 step programs know and use calling and reaching out at any time of night and it's a loving and compassionate tool that is good for both parties. A lot of focus needs to be on teaching breathing exercises and using meditative tools. Several key nutrients will help. The person needs to have a pad and pen near the bed and write whatever they remember or what they feel and think.

9. Repetition compulsion and ritualistic behaviors - These are ok and will pass over time. The mind is just stuck in a mental grove. The yogic masters call this samskara. All of us have them. It a natural part of the persons healing and family members need to be patient and know they will not last forever. A difficult challenge is when the grove the mind is stuck in is the reliving the trauma. Keep in mind that in the brain and emotional body all traumas are connected, no matter when it occurred in the life cycle. I was taught by my master, Swami Satchidanada, that sitting and learning to calm the mind and engaging in breath work

would help me develop a witness state where I was not in denial, but also not the event, that I was deeper than the event and that the soul or spirit cannot be traumatized, just the body, mind, and emotions. The swami went into a cave in the north of India for one year alone to face all his samskaras. Swami g was successful, but myself, I am not headed for any cave anytime soon. I did get to visit his cave several years ago, while on a journey thru India and it was pretty fascinating. I was surprised when our group sat and meditated for what we thought was about a half hour only to find out we were in the cave for four fours. Although it was a magical place, you don't need a cave to learn to help control your mind after a major hit. It is not hard to create your own safe place or to create an altar or table with your symbols that will remind you where you belong and that you are loved.

10. Loss of sexuality - It could be that the event created a loss of sexual desire, a huge thing in PTSD. This is a big loss for the person and their significant partner. I encourage all the people I work with to get some testing for estrogen and testosterone levels and also cortisol and some other things that can be tested. Any type of sexual abuse may drop levels drastically. Also, sex may have become something very different once you were violated. This a huge issue and will take time to heal. Time is the main healer and couples can be taught intimacy exercises that are not sexual. This is a good time to see if you have the ability to develop a spiritual practice. A very good time to stop self-judgment and begin the process of restoring love to yourself. PTSD prevents loving oneself and the love of a good friend, family members, and a therapist is going to be needed.

11. Anger - I saved this one for last because this is the one we see the most in any traumatized person or anyone with PTSD. They have

every right to be angry, yet it is going to spill out and there will be blow ups and the brain will be hijacked by anger and triggers the person did not know they had. Any minimizing of the event brings anger out fast. At times the person wants to act out on a physical level and hurt someone the way they have been hurt. Some want to hold on to anger as a form of protection and even feeling alive and not going into the numb state. Anger is not bad, it is human and there are many great ways to work with anger as it does flow up and out over time. Working in men's groups for so many years has taught me a lot of exercises to deal with anger. A huge 50 pound punching bag is hanging there, with boxing gloves for those that need to discharge anger. Over the years I have always seen the same thing once anger is discharged in men and that is loss and grief. Loss and grief are always the core feelings that anger is used to cover up. When the person moves thru the rage and anger and reaches the deep wound of grief in their hearts, they come home to who they truly are and healing begins in that moment. It is a beautiful thing to see, an honor and an opportunity for a giant shift in the PTSD process. I have been thrown across the room many times in groups, but I always land safely and unhurt, but joyful that movement is happening.

Clinical Approaches to Treatment of Trauma

Here are some of the ways that clinicians are treating traumas today in practice:

1. Metadata:
   a. This deals with the story or event and structure of the event, like a samsara in yogic thinking, it is the grove the trauma engraves in your mind and brain.

      b. Removing the metadata, where the brain stores memory and ending and changing the sensory inputs.

2. Trigger changing:

      a. Teaching the person a form of brain remapping to perceive the triggers in a different way.

      b. Looking at the triggers and letting go of the power the trigger holds over you. One way is changing the trauma into a super-stimulus that creates an anchor of safety.

      c. Where intense reactions from triggers are taken in in a different way and the brains perception changes over time and with work and help by a skilled therapist in brain remapping.

3. Neurofeedback:

      a. This is often used in remapping the brain and with trigger changing shifts. The client's head is wired to a laptop and clinicians have programs that can help in remapping. The therapist works with one over time and changes are made around key triggered events.

4. Resolution:

      a. Like a movie, change the scenes the brain sees, reverse the sequence thru hypnotic work, slow the time down and allow for resolution during the feeling of the event.

      b. NLP uses this a lot and finds useful.

5. Timeline:

      a. A timeline is about trying to change the story, can try working with it in reverse and turn the story inside, out.

6. Hypnotic Regression:

      a. Using emotional kinesthetic, guiding one thru the sequence of traumatic events while seeing new outcomes based on old events.

7. Deactivating the trigger:
   a. Time distortion and seeing the trigger as gone, over, done and one that can no longer hurt you today and then adding a new outcome to the event, one you can live with and be okay with.
8. EMDR:
   a. With a skillful therapist who has studied and worked using this method, one can reverse the brains pathways and remap the brain around painful memories of events.
   b. Therapist can also bring in love, light, and support when the client reaches space of big triggers and know there are not alone.
   c. Also allows one to pause during the work and often recall things stored in the brain that they did or were not able to recall, as it comes up, it gets dealt with.
9. Release work:
   a. When the anger level is huge, a punching bag can be used to release anger, grief, loss and other feelings around the vent that are buried.
   b. The work can also be done in a group with other people who have been thru traumas in their life and understand what one is dealing with.
   c. Psychodrama often brings up traumas and release can be done when brought up.
10. Emotional Freedom Tech (EFT): EFT is used a lot now. Tapping is one form of EFT and there are others that help:
    a. Spinning feelings:
       i. Voices and core feelings arise in a safe space and spin until the core one is used to move thru the event.

ii. Help create change in the emotional being, which impacts brain chemistry.

b. Havening and tapping:

i. Based on Callahan's work and Ruden, the client is taught to tap on energy spots in the body that have to do with release and remapping the brain images.

ii. Exercise may start with the trauma or event, but bring good energy and love into self.

iii. The healing aspects and ability to heal one's self is a big part of tapping. The ritual is also good for calming things down and shifting the feelings and brain activity to healing.

iv. Tapping is believed to be helping in also remapping the brain and must be practiced a few times a day to have a therapeutic effect. The picture from the amygdala may be revealed and that image can change with tapping. I have seen this often.

c. Yoga practice:

i. Any form of Yoga practice will bring the mind, body, and spirit together and during the Hatha form the body often releases what it has held on to for some time. Often the person may not have control over this and may cry during yoga class. I have had this happen to myself when I taught yoga in many situation's over the years. Often I taught in institutions and perhaps the people were more ready or in touch to let go. The asanas in Hatha are made to shift and help the body let go of what it does not need to carry any longer.

ii. There are also other yoga practices that may help, but I would only use them with a mentor or teacher who has been thru this dealing with trauma. Jnana Yoga is the practice of "Who Am I." Am I this event that I had little control over? Am I this body and brain that may have been impacted by the event? This practice was made by Ramana Maharshi, a great saint in India who taught this to all his students. He helped them develop a witness state where they could witness the trauma, the mind and the body's reactions, without engaging in the story or charges that the event creates. Thru deep meditation, one would reach a clear, calm and somewhat serene space and from that space, all could be witnessed without emotion. The brain could also be taught to become calm and accepting around the event, once the charge was gone. Again, this is for long time students of yoga with a skillful teacher and not meant to do on your own.

d. Somatic healing:

i. Using deep breath work, a trained therapist relaxes your body and helps you reach a semi trance like state where deep breathing stays throughout the processes. Images may come up and sensations from the body may come up surrounding events from the trauma. One needs to be in a place and try to be willing to let go. As they come up, the triggers are dealt with in a loving way, accepted, and felt in a gentle way.

ii. Time takes its time. No rush and sessions will build to a place of trust and release over time. The therapist will often write down things if they interact with the client as they may in some sessions. It is thought that the amygdala will release during somatic sessions.

Observation has taught me that when it comes to trauma each brain and emotional person is different. It is a process to learn and see what works best for each individual. Talking about the event too soon after the event at times will not work. It is almost like the brain is on lock down and needs to protect itself and survive. The person may just need more time before they begin the therapy and healing process. Pushing one into treatment too fast when they are not ready is not a good thing based on how the brain works. It is also important to understand that all traumas are linked in the brain and emotional body. They are not separate. It is almost if joined by a string and dealing with one event will often unleash other buried events that are stored in the amygdala. A person can begin to speak or work around one recent event and suddenly be back in something long forgotten from childhood that is coming up for the first time just now. One must be very gentle with this, it is totally out of the person's control.

Finally, what is our attitude? How do we deal with challenges? What are our connections in life, our spirituality, our commitment to service and helping those in need? There is no limit to the amount of love you can feel. That choice is up to you. Love changes everything!!!

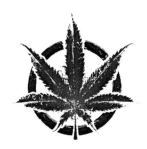

Toxic Marijuana Syndrome (TMS)

The Briarcliff Institute for Recovery and Development is involved with a study of young people ages 16 to 25 who are Marijuana addicts (as indicated by chronic marijuana use for the past two years).

Here is a profile including the symptoms of the illness, possible causes, and treatment plans for TMS:

Symptoms of TMS:

1. Academic problems
2. Peer problems, co-ed relationship concerns, and inability to maintain romantic relationships for extended periods of time.
3. Anger, irritability, conflict with parents, short fuses, and hi-jacking quickly into emotional states with no Pre Frontal Lobe intervention available.
4. An extreme state of apathy, lethargy, and an inability to motivate.
5. Shifts in level of communication skills.

6. Pre-existing conditions that have escalated due to marijuana use such as anxiety, depression, and active ADHD.

7. Failure to launch, leave home, move into the world, stuck in time and recycling themes and issues.

8. Self-esteem issues that have become extremely toxic and are not responding to treatment interventions.

9. Any trauma experienced (like loss of a grandparent or auto accident) is not felt, processed, or supported by existing brain chemistry functions.

10. Sudden returning from college and dropping out and loss of focus on the future.

11. Lack of passion in almost all areas of life, including sexuality.

12. Not responding to any interventions of medications due to receptor site impact.

13. Frequent headaches and respiratory problems with no response to medical interventions.

We realize many young people struggle with these symptoms and that they are often a reflection of adolescent development, but most have not ingested the toxins these TMS youths have.

Causes of TMS:

1. Metal toxicity from using one-hitters, bongs and pipes made from glass, plastic and metals, thus inhaling fumes that are toxic along with THC. Toxicity enters but cannot be removed without proper methylation treatment.

2. Fumes become highly toxic if coper, lead, aluminum, titanium screening is used

3. Inhaling toxic residue from pesticides, fertilizers, and laced marijuana that remain in the fat soluble cells in the brain and

body, causing shifts in brain chemistry due to the long acting presence of THC.

4. Ingestion thru inhalation of Butane from highly 80% potent Dabs that have become extremely popular.

5. Major psychological issues due to the unbalanced state of Methylation in the body and brain.

6. Possible Zinc deficiency.

7. Impact on brain and emotions, due to laced marijuana with K2, Spice or Sonic boom or any synthetic form of THC, which are easily available on the internet. Thus many unknown chemicals remain in the myelin sheath long after use stops.

8. Use of medical marijuana that has not been grown organically and may contain soil and environmental toxicity, along with illegal, high grade pesticides. This young person may be confident that the marijuana is pure, organic, and safe but is often wrong in their assumptions.

9. The rise of gangs tinkering with marijuana to compete with medical marijuana may contribute to ingestion of known and unknown substances (We have tested kids for THC and they were surprised to find ecstasy, opiates, meth, and PCP in their saliva).

10. Soil samples taken from both medical marijuana and street marijuana, like kush have shown high amounts of mold, fungi, higher levels of zinc not meant for human consumption. Some soils tested revealed toxic levels of copper in them. (Tests done by the Los Angeles city attorney found dangerously high levels of the pesticide Bifethrin. This is 1600 times higher than it should be and this was medical marijuana. Other studies found high levels of Diazinon, Pormethrin, and paclobutrazol)

11. Frequent relapse while in treatment and failure to recover after inpatient treatment centers, where brain chemistry is not dealt with.

Treatment options:

- Dr. Wilson and the removal of metal, pesticide and butane toxins thru his program.
- Methylation products used under the supervision of Systemic Formulas, a Nutrient company.
- Nutrient interventions at Briarcliff Institute with supervision and training from Dr Wilson.
- Detoxification programs such as Hippocrates Institute.

The young people in our study are now in the process of testing to confirm toxicity and will be involved in restoration treatment.

Many young people come to The Briarcliff Institute for Recovery and Development (BIRD) in various stages of weed use along the spectrum. Some are clearly recreational users who are young and experimenting with weed. They have not used too long or too often. This group tend to engage in treatment early. Yet there is another population we see, a large population of young people between the ages of 15-25 who have become chronic weed users. They often smoke daily or several times a day. We have been working with these young people for many years. They come to us for a variety of reasons, but they share many things and have many similarities.

I began to see a pattern of serious chronic weed use years ago. After engaging in treatment with our staff many stopped or reduced their use significantly. The majority of cases involved family therapy and consistent family engagement with the treatment team. Various services were offered, but never forced upon them. Although several of the cases in the 15-25 age group came to us in resistance, minimizing their drug use, we were ultimately able to engage them. We became skillful in making them feel safe at the institute. We refrained from judgment and looking at them like clinical cases but instead as real human beings who deserved to be treated with respect, compassion, and kindness. The goal in the beginning of treatment was around what was holding them back in life. It seemed like many were not evolving.

Knowing that many of the TMS symptoms mirror a lot of adolescent and young adult behaviors it became clear to me that TMS, as an illness or state of altered brain chemistry, body chemistry and functioning, would have to become validated. It also would need to be differentiated form these other typical adolescent and young adult behaviors. During my training at the Alliance for Addiction Solutions (ASS), I had learned a significant amount about metal toxicity and the importance of the balance of proper myth elation. One of the top doctors in the USA in metal toxicity, Dr. Wilson, provided a great interview for this book. In addition, Dr. Walsh from the Walsh institute, Dr. Morris and Dr. Tipps from a large Nutrient company in Utah, called Systemic Formulas, assisted in providing information for this book. In fact, after providing some initial information Dr. Morris and Dr. Wilson decided to work on our TMS study as a consultant.

Thru Dr. Wilson's program we had the great pleasure of working with Ms. Kathleen Korda. Her role was to test the young people utilizing hair samples to test for metal toxicity and nutrient balancing and get a better understanding of their levels of zinc, magnesium, copper, potassium as well as other chemicals. Dr. Wilson was responsible for supervising all of the testing in the first round of tests. The goal of this study was to prove that TMS is a serious illness and health threat to people of all ages, specifically young people. I was deeply impressed by all of the doctors at Systemic Formulas who gave their time willingly and free of charge to the Briarcliff Institute to pursue what we all felt was important research to help our kids. Dr. Wilson was even kind enough to offer to train me in metal toxicity and the removal of toxic metals and balancing the brain and body chemistry of our kids. He felt it would be important to have an in house treatment protocols. The unwavering support of these doctors reminded me of the old saying, "when the student is ready, the teacher appears." I should say that Dr. Wilson is not a big proponent of Medical Bud and expressed his concerns about any level of toxicity that could reach patients who were already ill. Dr. Wilson also validated my instincts and hypothesis about what may be found in the testing rounds. The doctor had strong feelings around how weed was impacting the brain chemistry and functioning of young developing brains. He, along with other individuals from Systemic Formulas, were very optimistic in that we would be able to remove the toxins and balance these kids out via the use of nutrient therapy.

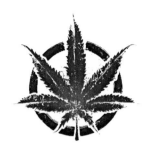

RESEARCH ON WEED

In this chapter, I will present some of the most current research on weed conducted by the scientific community and some other sources. There is not a lot of funding for weed research and until recently there was even less for medical weed. Surely Israel is way ahead of us as you will see in the chapter, The Israel Connection. I was curious as to why there was so little investment by our government on a substance that is being used by 12 million people, most under the age of 25. My guess is that weed has been so integrated into our culture. It is legal in many states and is often seen as a harmless gateway drug that may or may not lead young people to harder drugs. In addition, I would hypothesis that most young people would not want to be in a study involving weed unless they were given some good bud and paid. I myself am amazed that our small place, The Briarcliff Institute for Recovery and Development (BIRD), was able to get our young clients committed to the study. I was blessed with having the most incredible kids and they were hanging around long enough to pull it off.

The following is a list of interesting research conducted on marijuana. I will reference many of these studies throughout the book. I will save my comments for the end of the chapter.

1. Chemical Research in Toxicology published a great piece in June, 2014 emphasizing that smoking bud has proven the potential to trigger DNA damage. This falls under the topic of Epigenetics and Weed and you can read that chapter for more information on this.

2. A study conducted at The University of Leicester showed that weed would change molecules in DNA and alter molecules within the cells themselves. Some of these changes, the study claims, has the potential to trigger cancer. Specifically, the chemicals they found in the weed included aramatic hydrocarbons, aceteldehyde, napthalene, and benzanpyrene. Researchers used a mass spot metrics device in a lab setting.

3. An article from The Medical Press (2014) states that research has shown when controlling for major medical conditions, heavy THC use alters Neurotoxicity and causes alterations in the teen brain effecting development. The results include impairment in thinking, poor educational outcomes, symptoms of chronic bronchitis, as well as increased risk of psychotic disorders in those that are predisposed.

4. From the same source, Medical Press (2014), research found that brain imaging of regular weed users had shown significant changes in the brain structure. Among adolescents, abnormalities in the grey matter of the brain associated with intelligence were found in 16-19 year olds who had increased their weed use in the past year. These findings remained even after researchers controlled for things like prenatal drug exposure, developmental delays, and learning disabilities. The same article

went on to say that medical weed had much higher levels of THC in them than other strains of weed. The research had shown that frequent use of high potency weed can increase risk of acute and future problems with depression, anxiety and mental illness may be moderated by how often weed is used and its potency. The study showed that teens had a much more accepting attitude towards using medical weed and thus, were using it more frequently.

5. The Science Daily (2014) reported that a Loyola University Health System study found that more teens smoke weed than tobacco and have no stigma attached to their use, even though the article claims that weed is an addictive substance. The article also states that marijuana use is the number one addiction being treated in teen treatment centers. Many teens are using weed to manage depression and anxiety.

6. A recent study reported in The Journal of Neuroscience (4/16/14) conducted MRIs on 18-25 year olds who smoked weed at least once a week. Results indicated that these individuals had significant brain changes from those who did not smoke weed at all. The Nucleus Accumbens, a part of the brain involved in the reward process, was larger and altered in its shape and structure. The study went on to say light and moderate weed use will cause change in brain anatomy. Another aspect of the study focused on the part of the brain called the Amygdala, which plays a major role in emotion and how we process the stimulation coming in from the outside world. The study showed a difference in twenty users showing abnormalities in that part of the brain. The research was funded by the National Institute of Drug Abuse.

7. Schizophrenia Bullitin-12/16/14. This study was able to show that weed related brain abnormalities are correlated with a poor

working memory performance and tend to look very similar to schizophrenia related brain abnormalities. Researchers claim that changes in the brain structure may lead to changes in the way the brain will function. This study showed that the younger the individuals were when they started chronically using weed, the greater impact it had on their brains. The study claimed that the brain changes remained years after stopping the weed use. There also is a connection with the fact that if someone has had a family history of schizophrenia, they are increasing their risk of developing the disorder by abusing weed.

8. The Science Daily (4/11/11) reported on a study from the University of Western Ontario looking at how weed affects the way the brain processes emotional information. Weed impacts naturally occurring receptors in the brain called cannabinoid receptors. Those receptors are also found in the amygdala part of the brain responsible for emotion and also the fight or flight instinct. It dramatically increased the activity patterns of neurons in a connected region of the brain called the pre frontal lobe cortex, controlling both how the brain received emotional information of incoming sensory information and stimulus and the strength of memories associated with the emotional experience. The study is claiming that heavy weed use impacted the cannabinoid system of receptor sites in those brain regions distorting the emotional relevance of incoming sensed information which in turn can lead to side effects like paranoia. The development and discovery of the brains new patterns and pathways and these cannabinoid sites has great implications in developing pharmacological compounds that could block or modify these brain pathways and perhaps a way can be found to block these psychotic episodes. It may also help those who

suffer with PTSD (already being proven in Israel as seen in The Israeli Connection chapter).

9. Science Daily - Society of Nuclear Medicine (6/13/11) is an article that deals with more research of the cannabinoid receptors in the brain. The entire body has receptor sites that have a wide variety of functions. Two known ones are the CB1 and the CB2. CB1 is involved in the central nervous system, while CB2 is involved in the function of the immune system in stem cells and the circulatory system. Researchers are starting to study these two major receptor sites and are hopeful that medicines can be developed to treat cancer and other disorders.

10. The Journal of Studies on Alcohol and Drugs (8/15/14) reported on a study that shows that teens who are having a hard time managing their moods and experience frequent negative states of being will attempt to shift those feelings by smoking weed. One of the challenges here is that the teen will start to feel better with the weed, but then these same issues will resurface, but in a stronger and more powerful way. The study states that weed will also lower anxiety when it is smoked, but also return in a more powerful way once the effects of the weed have worn off.

11. In a study conducted by The Institute of Science at The University of Toronto the use of single photon emission computerized tomographic showed that after smoking weed activity was stimulated in the dopamine D2 receptor site and that the firing of dopamine was decreased by 20%, while there was an increase of dopaminergic activity. This study says that there may be an explanation for the increase and that it is linked to the psychoactive effects of weed on young people's brains and will impact those that are vulnerable. It also links a possible

connection between cannabinoid and dopaminergic systems in the brains reward pathways.

12. Alternatives for Alcoholism: Marijuana and its effects. This piece provides a comprehensive understanding of weed's effect on young people's brains. A neurotransmitter called endocannabinoid is involved with producing another chemical for transport anandamide. Anandamide is a Sanskrit word that means "Bliss" or "Delight". The neurotransmitter works by dampening down the effects of other neurotransmitter's matter. This is called retrograde signaling because it slows everything down. The Endo Cs land on the major Gaba, serotonin, dopamine, and they inhibit their effects. Anandamide is like the brains natural weed. As in the case with all the neurotransmitters, any artificial substitute will stimulate the receptor sites and trigger a decrease in brain production. Weed causes the high levels of dopamine and Gaba to be released creating a euphoric effect. As long as the two receptor sites are firing and releasing the nice, good feeling chemicals and the anandamides is flowing it's all good, but eventually the brain responds and thus receptor site activity decreases. After a while of marijuana use Gaba and dopamine become depleted (Note: This is why The amino Gaba is used in BIRD's Nutrient Profile). Eventually, due to the process of re-uptake, our brains will want more and more of the weed or a higher level of the THC component that is in weed. Often young people consume more or stronger bud, thus depleting the neurons even more.

If we focus on this study you just read, you have learned about this amazing chemical, anandamide and its impact on feeling good. As the brain can produce its own endorphins by running, swimming, rock climbing and various other exercises, the brain has the ability to make us feel good. The Cbn1 and Cb2 receptor sites can also be activated thru natural events that make us feel good and produce this anandamide. Also proper nutrient balance in young people will lead them to feeling much better and less depletion over time. It is a gradual process quit different than the quick high that weed brings.

Lower levels of Gaba, dopamine, serotonin and other receptor sites will have a huge impact on the brain chemistry. Add toxicity, poor eating habits, no exercise, and stress and you begin to see a lot of things develop. The most common results we are seeing include depression, anxiety, loss of motivation, insomnia, poor levels of self-esteem, and some hopelessness. Many of these symptoms can be seen in the TMS profile. THC often attaches itself to the fatty acids cells and can linger in them for a long time. Clients often fail a drug test for THC six weeks after stopping use of weed. Most young people don't get enough fatty acids in their diets unless they are supplementing with nutrients. Also today, the lower fat diet is more popular in general and more and more kids are becoming vegetarians or not eating as much meat as they once did because their parents have made a lot of dietary changes. As depletion of the brain unfolds and toxicity raises, all due to chronic weed use, it becomes an epigenetic event and a personal crisis for children and their parents.

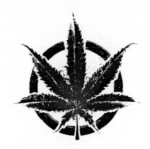

EPIGENETICS AND BUD

What is Epigenetics and how could it have anything to do with using weed? This chapter will tackle this question and hopefully provide a whole new understanding around this relatively new field.

Very simply, Epigenetics is the new field of study that looks at how environmental factors impact the genes and our DNA. It also looks the impact of environmental factors over generations in families where certain illnesses may be handed down from one generation to another. Epigenetics is very similar to what the founder of family therapy, Murray Bowen looked at. Bowen was concerned with family beliefs, attitudes, mental disorders, addictions, and anything that repeated from one generation to the next. Bowen called this The Multi-Generational Transmissions Process. As a young family therapist and videographer at a family therapy training institute, I was very fortunate to spend some time with Bowen and watch his work closely. He believed that if one generation did not deal or fix an issue it would get handed down to the next generations growing stronger as it kept getting handed down.

When we apply Bowen's ideas to Epigenetics, we see many similarities. Looking at the drastic changes in our environment over the past several years we have to consider possible toxins in the environment, if they have been ingested, and if they remain in our systems, our genes, our coding and DNA impacting who and what we are. Are these environmental changes negatively or positively impacting our makeup? Are we able to alter these changes or are they permanent? Consider an individual ingesting toxic chemicals from weed, a plant that had been altered by chemicals like pesticides, fertilizers, metals or other additives in the soil it was harvested in. Or if the said individual ingesting weed was using butane, hot glass pipes, copper filters, titanium metal pipes, aluminum, plastic bongs, toxic water in bongs, or laced weed. Our brains can be significantly impacted by these chemicals causing dysfunctional behavior patterns. There dysfunctional behavior patterns ultimately impact the family system. Just as Bowen described, over generations certain traits become toxic in families. Our testing has revealed that over time many forms of weed and how it is consumed also has become toxic.

In biology, Epigenetics is the study of cellular and physiological traits that are not caused by DNA sequence. Epigenetics deals with long term alterations in transcriptional potentials of a cell or group of cells or in genes and DNA factors. Changes in gene expression or cellular phenotype of epigenetics may have other causes. Epigenetics looks at the balance of metals in the brain and having proper methylation levels for good brain functioning. Our focus here is looking at how the chemicals added to our environment are causing changes on cellular levels. We already know that chemical toxins can affect neuron and receptor site activity. As previously discussed, often times an individual smoking weed is ingesting high levels of copper, mercury, and cadmium. After weed use has stopped, the impact of toxicity may not go away and brain functions may not be fully restored without intervention. This all depends on the levels of toxicity and how the person is integrating the nutrients coming into their systems.

Chronic weed use may elicit a sedamentated state with long lasting changes of intracerebral gene transcription. Evidence from animal studies have started to assimilate itself into mediating roles of epigenetic mechanisms. A recent study conducted at the School of Medicine at Mt. Sinai focused on human genes by the transcription factors. Proteins that bind to specific DNA sequences influence the function of genes. Genes can be altered by exposure to chemicals and also stressors resulting in the genes becoming more susceptible to addiction. When the researchers introduced synthetic transcriptions factors called Zinc proteins or Zinc fingers into a single gene in the Nucleus Acumens, the part of the brain that is closely associated with maintaining the production of the chemical dopamine and serotonin, they saw significant changes in that area. These findings indicated more sensitivity with drug interaction activity. Weed is impacting epigenetics. Epigenetics can define how the information in the cells are expressed and then how they impact and alter brain chemistry. When an organism grows and develops, carefully orchestrated chemical reactions will activate and de-activate parts of the genome at strategic times and in specific locations. Our brains were not made with the capacity to eliminate metals, most likely because we were never meant to allow toxins and metals to cross the brain barrier.

The primary psychoactive component in weed is tetrahydrocannabinol (THC). It is believed that it exerts its psychological effects via the disruption of normal cannabinoid receptor sites. It sends signals into the brain that elicits long term molecular and cellular changes in the brains of humans and of those of studies done with mice, predominately impacting neuronal signaling in brain structure in the Acumen's and Hippocampus. Duration of marijuana use as well as the age in which one engages in use plays the greatest role on the impact on brain development. If you recall from the previous chapters, between the ages of 14 and 26 the brain has the greatest growth. There is no doubt in my mind that epigenetics is impacting that period of growth in the chronic weed users we have seen and tested.

Dr. Walsh, of the Walsh Institute, is one of the world's leaders in methylation and epigenetics. He answered many questions for me during a webcast that the Alliance for Addiction Solutions (AAS) hosted. Dr. Walsh has also presented a study where he was able to go into a prison and test copper levels in crack addicts. What he found was that although many had not used for some time, the copper levels remained high, thus causing many more aggressive incidents. Unstable levels of copper in the brain is connected to violence and aggression. The copper in these research participants did not come from the drug crack, but from the screening used in glass pipes to smoke the crack. In his excellent book "Nutrient Power," Dr. Walsh writes on epigenetics and brain functioning, "Healthy mental functioning requires a proper level of synaptic activity at the receptor sites for dopamine, norepinephrine, serotonin, Gaba, endorphins, and other neurotransmitters." He states that proper synaptic activity depends on the following factors; the amount of neurotransmitters produced in brain cells, the amount of neurotransmitters lost by diffusion or by reacting to chemicals ingested, and the availability of transporters that will return synaptic transmission back into the original brain cells for re-uptake process. (Re-uptake is greatly affected by consistent drug use of any kind.)

Epigenetic research has identified several other kinds of nutrients that have the potential for improving and repairing brain chemistry. SSRIs, such as Prozac, are no longer our only option. SSRIs are used by psychiatrists to help young people raise their serotonin levels. There is a strong indication that they will not work as well in young people who chronically use bud. There is research indicating nutrient protocols can change the brain. I have failed to see SSRIs work in any kid who uses weed at least four times a week. The other aspect is that the client, being young and not sure of the doctor, may not always tell the truth or be totally authentic about the level of their use for fear of disclosure to their parents.

Some new studies using epigenetics are exploring and showing that gene expression and brain chemistry can be severely altered by too many toxic chemicals from the environment. Methylation and the proper metal levels are responsible for a young and old person's mental health. High levels of histamine indicates under methylation, while low levels of histamine indicate high methylation. Under methylation in mental health looks like obsessive and compulsive disorders, very strong willed and resistant to change, competitive, ritualistic behaviors, high libido, addictions, depression and perfectionism. While over methylation in mental health often manifests as high anxiety, increased fears, low libido, sleep disorders, multiple food and chemical sensitivity, antihistamine intolerance and adverse reactions to the SSRI meds.

For those interested in learning more about all this, Dr. Welsh's book is excellent and not hard to read. Dr. Welsh was too busy to consult on our project but our two doctors, Dr. Wilson and Dr. Morris are also experts in this field and you can refer to their chapters to see their input on what they found in the BIRD study.

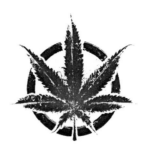

ADDICTION RISK

Some young people just seem to be more prone to risky behaviors. These are the types of kids that love on the edge activities growing up. They will sled into streets, climb trees that they are unable to get down, and pick up their parents' gin and tonic and gulp it down. Give one of these kids a skateboard and watch, they will be on their edges quick, and they will bruise. A child like this not only has difficult slowing down their bodies but also struggles to slow down their brain. They may have increased levels of dopamine. Some of us are just born with excessive or deficient levels of certain chemicals like dopamine, serotonin, or endorphins. It's just brain chemistry and nobody's fault. We will discuss this in greater detail in the chapter on epigenetics.

Often, these kids get labeled as "bad kids." Parents often, far too often, see these types of children as a bad influence on their own children. I hear this a lot from parents and challenge them in their thinking and belief systems. To have a young child judged and then to try to eliminate them from your child's life is very limited thinking to me. It is my belief that people should learn before they judge. It is important for parents to know their own children and what they bring to the dance because there are no perfect beings out there. It is all for growth, learning, and the child's evolution. Based on my experience, I have found that children are better off experiencing life rather than being sheltered and thus not having some of the things in life that will challenge them in how they want to be and what choices they want to make. They may end up saving another kids life because kids without limits and no brakes in their brains need slower, more thoughtful kids around. Compassion is a choice in life!

A low dopamine child will spend hours on internet gaming, sports, girls, and will be more prone to try substances as a way of waking up their brain and feeling alive. The main thing is that they need to feel alive. They don't want to feel flat and disconnected. They want to move and do things that will wake their spirits and brains up. They will need to be stimulated. These are the types of children who are likely to love stimulant drugs. They may also be attracted to weed. They typically like the feeling of things being intensified, colors brighter, sounds sharper, and thoughts that move and have rhythm to them. Weed is like music to their brains. THC will work its way to the dopamine receptor site and if it is low, it will create the illusion that it is increasing. Weed works very well on dopamine receptor sites. Most children with ADHD are drawn to weed because it will often work in reverse and calm the overheated brain down. The brain creates the energy of needing something. Individuals tend to look at the young person choosing to smoke marijuana as a choice. Perhaps we need to look at brain chemistry and our ability or inability to control it.

As a young child, I was a serious risk taker. I would climb the highest tree and the fire department would have to be called to get me down. Once, at age 13, I skateboarded with a tow rope attached to a mini bike some kid in my neighborhood had built. An hour later I found myself in the ER getting bones reset. Not even a month later I tried to cross the Long Island sound on a tube. I never considered how this would impact my poor mother who was afraid of water, despite always living near water. The coast guard was called, police, harbor patrol, even the fire department. The firemen were getting to know me. I felt bad because I knew they had real things to deal with and lives to save. I was cooking hot dogs on some rocks with a group of homeless individuals living in a shack out on an abandoned island, the guard came upon me. Right away, they dug in. "Hey kid! Don't you know your mother thinks you drowned and you're dead!" Upon returning with the coast guard there were tons of people, police, etc. lined up on the shoreline waiting for me. I asked the guy on the boat if he could drop me somewhere else! The funny thing is my mom did not react to me as if I had just died. No way! She was mad! Crazy angry! I was in trouble once again. I could go on and on with stories similar to this one. Eventually I got a bad reputation. Some mothers would not let their kids have me over or come over. Somehow we always found a way to get together, ignoring them. The thing is that I was deeply liked, even loved by so many, but was considered to be kind of crazy!

Many risk seeking kids will smoke weed early. Starting as early as 12 or 13 years old. It is very common for kids to come to treatment already addicted to weed by 13. Things are moving much quicker in our world. Risk taking kids do not think when a hit of smoke is passed to them. It is like an automatic response. It feels good. They will act immediately and think about it later. Unfortunately, most kids will not share with their parents that they have been trying weed. They may feel they have let their parents down and failed them somehow. They may have guilt, even shame. Some simply just will not care. Some will have come from parents who smoked themselves, thus making it totally acceptable for the child to try it too. Some kids will have gotten their first bag of weed from their parents stash. Hey Parents... If you think you can hide the fact that you enjoy smoking weed from your kids, just remember, they will see right thru you to the place you stashed it.

Ideally it would be great to identify the risky kids and work with their wiring and personality early, before the brain moves towards cravings in other more harmful ways. I wish, I could have done that myself. Years later, after doing this work for a while, I did some brain mapping and neurofeedback and was not surprised to find I had a brain deficient in both dopamine and endorphins. Ouch!! Brain mapping and neurofeedback technologies are now available, however there is debate over whether Brain Mapping is 100% accurate. I have seen amazing results with Brain Mapping and some very good work with neurofeedback for risk related addiction.

I feel I would be remise if I don't mention gaming as part of this conversation. There is little difference in the brain of a gamer and that of an individual using substances. There are many parallels. Parents often ask what the right amount of time is for a 16 year old to be playing internet and video games, interactive or not. To help with this question, we need to understand that studies have shown that gaming will cause dopamine and other chemicals in the brain to shift and change. Research also indicates that children become easily addicted to gaming. This can be problematic as it often goes unaddressed as it is socially acceptable. I often speak with parents who tell me their child is playing up to 6 hours a day. But not alone they say, they have friends over or are online. Parents somehow feel that if peers are involved, it is a "social activity" and it is okay. It is important for parents to understand that these kids can not pull back from these games on their own. They will play for several hours. I have seen it. The brain is totally consumed. The personality, the mind, body, and spirit are only engaged in the goals of the game.

The inability to regulate ones behavior is always a sign that parents may want to think about intervening. I ask parents to try and begin with kids regulating their time to an hour and a half a day, two hours on weekends. It's not a bad thing for receptor sites to get stimulated. It's over stimulation and burn out that we want to watch for. It is also important to watch for avoidance of doing other important developmental things and making gaming the only priority. Human connectedness is imperative for all human beings. It feels good and feeds the brain. Love will always feed every aspect of us. It knows no bounds. It is hard to find true connectedness and love in gaming.

On a final note, when your child starts asking you about your own drug use when you were younger, make sure you throw a question back at them. Why do you want to know? You can assume something is in the undertow in their life. Risk takers also seem to love money, gambling, and what I would just call juice, being in action. My advice to parents is to stay connected to your kid and their finances. Younger kids should not be walking around with wads of cash. Money creates juice, juice turns into a rush, the rush is liked and that moves towards addiction.

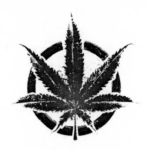

ATTENTION DEFICIT HYPERACTIVITY DISORDER (ADHD) AND BUD

Over the years I have had a lot of clinical experience working with and treating young people who were diagnosed with Attention Deficit Hyperactivity Disorder (ADHD). One thing many of them had in common was that they like and used a fair amount of bud. I find children diagnosed with ADHD tend to be very descriptive. I believe this is a result of compensating for their lack of attention by developing their other senses. I relate to the ADHD child with heightened visual senses. I was a professional photographer prior to becoming a social worker and I saw the world in a very visual way. I believe this commonality between myself and the ADHD child helped when developing rapport as they felt I actually understood how they process the world and how their minds worked. I am going to describe their experiences with bud during early experimentation stages or let's call it "recreational use" through my own personal perspective:

1. Weed was great for my mind and brain. I became so zoned in and focused and more sensitive to my environment. My mind definitely slowed down, but in a different way ADHD meds slowed me down. This felt more natural.

2. I was able to get thru situations better and even quicker with bud. I wouldn't get as distracted.

3. It finally felt like my mind had calmed down and that this may be what "normal" feels like?

4. I definitely felt it worked better at first than stimulant medication such as Adderall, Ritalin, Vyvanse, etc. Those took me out of my life and felt nasty.

5. I was able to get thru my homework more efficiently. My mother was always surprised when I was done. She didn't know I was blazing! (You're not going to tell her now. Are you?)

6. Although I noticed that bud affected my memory, I still felt I was tuned into and engaged in a much more productive way.

7. My mind did not wonder as much, except in math class (but we all know math is a waste of time).

8. My parents and siblings thought I was on a better path in life when I was smoking. They believed I was more focused and "grounded."

9. I could see or get a visual of the material the teacher was presenting. I love that my brain can do that! Can other kids to that? Do they? Do you?

Sounds to me like a wonder drug for ADHD kids! It is hard to know which component of the bud is making the most impact on the ADHD brain, tetrahydrocannabinol (THC) and cannabidiol (CBD) (explained in full in chapter on The Israeli Connection). There are at least 25 cannabis receptor sites in the brain and body, one of the components is most likely increasing dopamine and Gaba, but in a very different way than stimulants would. I would say that early recreational use, as described honestly by the clients I have met at BIRD is having a huge positive impact on the brain and ADHD.

Research as referenced in the Research on Weed chapter, has shown weed raises dopamine in early use. It will take brave organizations willing to put themselves out there saying they are thinking about medical marijuana for treatment of ADHD. We don't know in 10-20 years from now how medical marijuana will be used and for what conditions. Did we ever imagine we would be able to isolate the THC from the highly medicinal CBD? Did we ever think that sever, eight, and nine year old children would be getting strains of weed from Colorado that don't even have THC in them. These strains only contain CBD and eliminating seizures and helping epileptic's more than anything else has. Did we think a farm in Israel would isolate the many medicinal aspects of weed without the high? An O'douls beer for the weed smokers! Wild stuff! That Dr. Raphael Mechoulam (grandfather of weed research) would spend his whole life studying this THC plant. Something is definitely going on in that pin ball bouncing brain when weed hits it. The ball slows down. I have seen dozens of 15, 16, 17 year olds self-medicating with weed for ADHD. I could easily see hundreds of interviews with these kids if they could be honest and authentic. I strongly believe that science would benefit from more research on moderate early weed use with ADHD kids.

Now, let's look at the other side. Some of these self-medicaters are going to become addicted, daily users and some multiple daily users, as their bodies develop tolerance of the drug. They started with trying to treat themselves and many moved into the progression of addiction. Some lose the power of choice. They hate their ADHD meds, want to make their parents happy, want to be successful in a demanding school setting, and want to be able to follow a conversation with a nice look-ing girl or guy. They find themselves on the spectrum as chronic users, then things begin to shift and change. Their parents catch them or a sibling smells the smoke on them. The brain begins to shift and change as dopamine does not raise sharpening their focus as it once had but now drops significantly making their attention and focus much worse. Focus gone, motivation wanes, attention goes, some get apathetic, some just give up and call themselves "stoners." Sad! They were just trying to make their parent's happy and live a more grounded life. No? A tolerance does not take long to kick in with weed because the brain is a smart place. It was not made by some fool! Whoever designed that baby knew their stuff.

As tolerance builds, some ADHD kids will shift to dabs, wax, but-ter or other substances. Much more potent types of marijuana. The kind of substance that gets a person so wasted they can't function nor-mally. With use of these stronger substances, memory becomes a ma-jor problem. Even simple attention takes a lot more work. The whole brain chemistry shifts. Dopamine goes down and Gaba gets depleted.

I found a huge parallel in the work of Dr. Amen on ADHD. He lists the forms of ADD (now encompassed under the ADHD diagnosis in the DSM V) in his excellent book "Healing ADD." He speaks of short attention span, impulsivity, irritability and an inability to shift attention. Sounds a lot like TMS (Toxic Marijuana Syndrome). Dr. Amen speaks of "temporal lobe ADD." When the Temporal lobe is impacted, the kids have more instability, temper control, mood insta-bility, aggression, and memory and learning problems. These are the same symptoms we see in TMS from chronic weed users.

He has another profile called the "limbic ADD profile." Children that fit this profile have depression that comes and goes. This is a low grade type of depression with persistent ADD symptoms. There is even a form of anxious ADD where kids have symptoms of anxiety, fear, and nervous tension that does not get released and they begin to expect the worst. Sounds a lot like TMS!! I have been able to witness this progression in so many young people over time. Once a brain is wired for weed it works against most, not all. I've tried many interventions along the spectrum of weed addiction, but the client needs to become abstinent in order for us to treat and repair their brains. The biggest challenge in ADHD children is often motivation and/or low self-esteem. Surely some of these kids will need psychopharmacology and we are certainly not against that. However, in chronic weed users meds don't work due to blockages in the receptor site area and severe nutrient depletion. Weed is a very thick, dusty, and oily substance in the brain and if toxicity is involved, as it is in the majority we have tested, the receptor sites may or may not be receptive to medication. However, those young people we are successful with getting them to stop smoking realize that weed is not only making their ADHD worse, but also making them feel bad all of the time. Those young people respond well to Nutrient Treatment very quickly. They also respond to meditation, yoga, exercise, group therapy with other young people who are just like them. Some will attend good NA or AA meetings geared toward the younger population of users.

Our research study deals with toxins and brain chemistry fallout. Much more research needs to be done on marijuana use for ADHD. We need to commit to helping children stuck in the cycle of marijuana use and abuse. To see these children coming to BIRD with such low self-esteem and feeling like failures before their life has even begun is tragic and unacceptable.

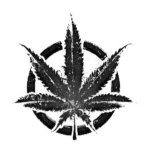

A WALK DOWN 7TH AVENUE

It is a beautiful warm May evening as I stroll down 7th Avenue in New York City. Walking past the cages, the famous NYC mecca of street ball, I have the incredible feeling of being alive. I spent much of my youth on these streets and I know the area well. As I walk around Greenwich Village I notice a lot of changes. However, after all of the time that has past many things have stayed the same such as the sweet smell of weed in the air. I am just a block or two away from the famous Washington Square Park where, just as it was fifty years ago, the walkers will hear the calls of loose joints.

My mission tonight is to check out some smoke shops in the area. I count 15 in a 15 block zone. I stop into a couple shops and check out the products. Every pipe imaginable can be seen and bought. There is a variety of incredible glass small one hitter pipes, in a multitude of colors. They look like works of art. Every type of size and shape can be had. Plenty of metal pipes also made of lead, titanium, aluminum, wood, glass and something the counter person calls titanium two! "That's the best man!" he tells me, "A bit more expensive, but strong and easy to clean out." I check it out. It's heavy. Small enough for one to three hits depending on how you fill it.

I strike up a conversation with a young African American man, Mustiff. He tells me he's been selling pipes for years in this area. He explains that it is a profitable business because his primary consumer is a younger population who will buy anything. "We don't get many people your age in here." He tells me as he checks me out. Mustiff takes some time to school me on the pipes. He prefers glass because they are so attractive and artistic and kind of fun. Metal is the most efferent, in his opinion. We move from small pipes, to bongs, to huge glass pipes, vapors, and plastic. I am thinking that there has to be 5,000 pipes in the store. I am asking a lot of questions for an older dude who just wants to buy a pipe. At some point he asks me if I am going to buy anything. I tell him no, not today, just doing some research to which he queries, "what do you mean research man?" I tell the truth about writing a book about weed and young people and concerns about metals from hot pipes getting into the brain while smoking weed. "What do you mean man, these pipes are not for weed, we don't run with that here, they for tobacco only. Nothing in this shop is for weed. Now, if you're not buying anything you got to go man, you're bad for business." With that, I leave.

I check out another smaller shop and here I ask the counter guy if the wood pipes are treated with any chemicals because they all appear to be laminated to withstand high heat and not catch on fire. He tells me yes, but has no idea what type of lamination is on the small one hitters, which by the way, are very cheap like $5 tops. After too many questions about the wood treatment, he starts to also get agitated with me and demands to know why am I asking so many questions and not buying anything. "I don't smoke weed." I tell him. "I am just doing some research for a book I may write or may not." "Get out of here." He tells me. "These pipes are all for smoking tobacco, not weed and if you aren't buying, you're lying so go, bro." Dude has a way with words so I go.

I stroll down to John's pizza, the best you will find in that hood, and Ferrero's bakery, also the best (and while you are there ask my man Rocco for a cappuccino. I hang and chat for a while with Rocco about the village and how it was back in the day and what it's like now. He tells me that most young people just smoke on the street and don't try or need to hide it anymore. I have a lot of respect for Rocco. He makes the best cannoli for sure! New Yorkers are talkers and love to give their opinions if you will hang to listen. I learn a lot about the neighborhood. What I found most interesting was that any kid can get any type of pipe they want if they have the cash. Most are not concerned with what the pipes are made of and what metals they may contain. That a titanium two pipe was going for twenty-five bucks! The best of the best! Once again I am forced to ponder what happens when the metals get extremely hot and release. What do they release into the brains of the young people we work with at BIRD? I start thinking about glass pipes being made from sand and thinking what's in sand these days? Mercury, Oils? I start thinking about the copper and lead screens I saw and know that when copper gets hot and enters the brain thru smoking weed, it's not going to be good for the user. I have already learned thru my survey that many kids use one hitters most frequently. Glass and metal are the most popular and they also create the most fumes. This information only solidifies my desire to find a way, a good testing system, to find out exactly how these chemicals in the fumes impact the young brain. I start to think about how I am going to be able to pull that off. After all, I am only a Social Worker and Nutrient Therapist and clearly not a scientist. I don't even recall if I passed science in High School. I find comfort in Rocco and his incredible cannoli's and my mind moves on.

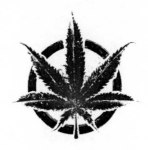

THE ISRAELI CONNECTION

While researching important information for this book, I discovered the Israeli connection. Israel leads the world on research around medical marijuana. They lead the world on developing systems of how the government, growers, and distributers can work together. Israel is setting examples for the world in growing a clean product free of toxic pesticides. When Doctors in the United States need information about using marijuana for medical purposes, they go to Israel for training and knowledge. Israel will also be the one to lead the world by becoming the first country with a successful government run pharmaceutical program and system for medical cannabis. True Bud! The amazing research and government funding to support research and treatment using medical weed in Israel is fantastic! It is exciting to see that marijuana can be put to good uses, with no toxicity and very little diversion to the street. There is a very different situation here in the states, where state and city programs have often spiraled out of control. They have put together a patchwork of constantly changing laws and taxes. We see daily explosions in Colorado from butane used for making dabs or hash oil. We see weed diverted to streets of every city. What we see is the gold rush. The amazing opportunity out west to make massive amounts of cash is irresistible.

Over 50 years ago Professor Raphael Mechoulam, nicknamed "The grandfather of pot," began research on marijuana. His work eventually awarded him the Rossschild Prize for outstanding research. Professor Mechoulam along with others working in the lab at the Weizmann Institute of Science in Rehovot, Isreal spent thousands of hours working hard on many aspects of using weed for medical purposes. The professor found Israel's Ministry of Health happy to assist in his work. By 1963, Mechoulam and his fellow researchers had found and begun to isolate the structure of THC. They were the first to discover CBD, or Cannabidiol, and isolate it. It is important to know that it is the THC in weed that gets you high, CBD does not. When isolated from THC, CBD has incredible medicinal potentials and qualities.

This chapter will illuminate some of the work going on in Israel, but it is also important to give the Stanley family, pot growers in Colorado, huge credit for their hard work on isolating CBD on their farm. The Stanley family developed a syrup out of marijuana known as Charlotte's Web, for a young child who was severely epileptic experiencing up to 50 seizures a day. Charlotte's Web contains CBD with barely readable levels of THC. With the regular use of this syrup extract the child is no longer considered epileptic. She was cured of her symptoms and able to live the life of a normal healthy child. Way to go Stanley brothers! I commend you for using the bud for good reasons, growing a clean product, and making a syrup extract for these epileptic kids.

Let's go back to Israel now. Israel's Government has been supporting a discreet expanding and very successful Medical Cannabis distribution center since 2008 known as "Mechkar." Israel has eight farms, distributing to over 12,000 patients, reaching high financial numbers far into the millions. Medical Weed is thriving in Israel under the strict control of the government. The Israeli government maintains an open and accepting attitude towards research projects geared toward assisting their sick countrymen and also helps out with the funding. Israel is involved in studies around using medical weed to help with PTSD (PTSD World, 10/2/13). The two professors researching this study are Mimi Peles and Dr. Allen Frankel from Telavi University. The Ministry of Health gave Dr. Frankel the green light to run clinical trials for those suffering PTSD. PTSD is a huge issue in Israel due to the constant threat of conflict, the actual threat of combat, and the Multi-Generational aspect of families having lived with everything from the holocaust to the Six Day War to present day conflicts. Over 200 individuals have participated in these studies, all carrying a diagnosis of PTSD, and all have been approved by the Ministry of Health to use the marijuana. One particular study, which is being conducted at the time I am writing *True Bud* involves 30 combat Veterans who have what is called Treatment Resistant PTSD. They will be studied before using the THC, then while using the THC, and then after to determine if their resistant PTSD improved as a result of their marijuana use. Although the study is not complete, Dr. Frankel has found that the medicinal THC helps his patients sleep which is often a huge problem with unresolved PTSD clients. It has also helped with lessening the impact of painful memories that arise decreasing their intensity and duration thus improving the veterans' quality of life.

According to the Jewish Journal (2013), a 2009 documentary film called "Prescribed Grass" was made in hopes of getting Israeli politicians to open their eyes to the needs of combat veterans with PTSD and other mental disorders. The documentary provided information on the benefits of marijuana research and medicinal use of the plant. The film shows some of the farming places in the country growing strains of weed. One such farm is called Tikun Olam. This farm has been able to grow special strains of cannabis that contained super high levels of cannabidiol, or CBD. These strains of cannabis were almost entirely void of THC, thus lacking that high producing feeling of euphoria. The hope at Tikun Olam is that their strain will be able to help in many medicinal ways without the feeling of being stoned. This same farm has also grown a strain of weed that has a 29 percent THC potency, which the farm claims is the highest ever recorded. They want to use this strain for cancer patients with pain and nausea. I imagine at some point we will see a strain war or competition evolve out of the medical weed industry to see who can make the most potent product? I would rather see a clean product. I care little about potency or strains, but more about toxicity and way of using the weed. It is important to note that the new highly potent form of bud called Dabs, Butter, Wax or concentrate has trumped the Israeli farm quite a lot. The Dabs are coming in at 80 to 90% potency of THC and most kids in high school know how to make it from the internet or by being taught by a friend. Please see the chapters dealing with Dabs and strains for potency levels and a great story by JP.

Back to the Israeli connection. THC is being used at the Sheba Medical Center in Israel to treat cancer patients. The patients inhale the weed thru a vaporizer that has been installed into the patients' hospital bed or room, depending on their mobility. If you can't get to the weed, it will get to you. One patient at Sheba is using cannabis in another very interesting way. This particular patient I am referring to is a holocaust survivor who had a stroke. The THC was helping him greatly with post stroke recovery. Surprisingly, the THC use began to assist him with many very painful childhood memories that went back to his being in a concentration camp. This 80 year old man began to feel better and lighter in life. Here, bud was a true blessing. Stories of

True Bud continue to amaze me. You will never hear me say that bud is good or bad or right or wrong. I will speak to the truth of true bud.

It is my belief and great hope that Israel will lead the world in the area of medical marijuana. Professor Ruth Gallily at Hebrew University conducts CBD research and confirms it is highly effective in its ability to help with inflammation. She said CBD is the best anti-inflammatory in the world. Another well-known Doctor from Hebrew University in use and research is Dr. Guzman. He is working on identifying the similarities between the newly discovered endocannabinoid system and the nervous system. The discovery of the CB1 and CB2 receptor sites has been huge for further research over there. CB1 is involved in the central nervous system, while CB2 is involved in the function of the immune system in stem cells and the circulatory system. Dr. Guzman is currently hard at work on his research on using cannabinoids to assist in tumor management. He has also looked at other uses for arthritis, auto immune diseases, diabetes, and even schizophrenia. Dr. Guzman has gone so far as to say that in some patients with very difficult cases the both forms of weed, THC and CBD, prolonged life and gave several patients hope.

In Israel, all cannabis users must get and have a license from the Ministry of Health. All patients who hold a card must receive training from the Ministry of Health around using the substance and the different strains. In addition they are charged $100 a month, weed of course included. Israel provides a clean, toxin free product. As you are reading this I am hoping that this country will have caught up on how well the medical marijuana industry is doing in Israel.

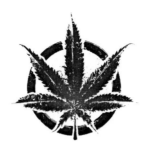

Strains and gains-Dabs so Fab?

I was young once! You could say I was around in the 60s. I saw a fair amount of the world and weed. Weed was abundant and it was hardly ever a problem to get. I had a friend who was a botany wiz who successfully grew his own weed. He was a botany wiz but eventually ended up dropping out of high school. He picked a secluded spot along the Long Island Sound. There were a lot of woods and I guess you could say that's where he attended most of high school. Most of the weed out on the street back then was from Mexico or Columbia. If you were lucky it was 7-12 percent THC. My man who grew obviously never tested his product, but it was much stronger than anything around and I think he was making more cash than the local Chevy dealership! I was the only one to ever visit the site and I am guessing he trusted me to not hit it up, which I never did. If we had gotten caught by the law, we would have gone away to jail for some time. Yet, the young brain does not compute these things and thankfully we were never caught.

I will tell you the truth, I did not care much for weed. My brain chemistry was just not wired for weed. On a trip to Morocco, I tried blond hashish and lost track of time, where I was, and only remember being chased down some ally by two big dudes with swords screaming, "get the Kennedy kid, we will sell him!" It did not take long for me to notice a connection between any substance use and mad crazy things unfolding in my world. I remember when Tai sticks came out and how much of a hit my friends took from those babies. I know they were not cheap, but they were much more potent than the Mexican stuff, which left many with headaches for days. In hindsight, it seemed all my Bud buddies always had headaches. Sensimillon, much stronger and again not my thing, became very popular and began to replace Tai sticks. This was right around the time when I left the little town along the Long Island Sound and did not return for several years, but that is a whole other story.

Things have moved along over the years and weed has evolved. I would say there are as many names and strains as types of alcohol. The majority of young people we see have a brand they like and seek out. What's popular these days? Kush, Sour, Deisel, Vanilla sky? All our young clients have no problem getting both medical weed from the West and edibles. One of the more popular edibles are jolly ranchers filled with around 15% THC. One article I came across claimed edibles gain potency as they move thru your system and that you end up much more messed up than smoking. The chronic users frequently ingest edibles and need a constant flow of weed coming all day.

The picture of potency looks very different with the new highly potent form of smokable THC called Dabs, Butter, Wax, and Concentrate. These products have an 80-90% potency and a much better chance of destroying your brain even further by ingesting butane and other not so good chemicals. Similar to some of the chemicals previously discussed, young people are ingesting Benzene, Hexane and other very toxic chemicals and impurities while smoking this concentrated THC. Young people will put wax on a nail made from lead or a pin made from aluminum in order to ingest the substance. There have also been many explosions in making these smokable forms of THC. But that is beyond the scope of this book. Although I was unable to find research on the impact of dabs, butter, etc. on brain chemistry, there was substantial literation indicating the health concerns around consuming these products. Some such concerns include the inhalation of dirty butane as well as inhaling or ingesting harmful contaminants that are basically unknown and infused into the concentrate during the extraction process. The extraction techniques used mirror those used in turning cocaine to crack as well as the process in Meth labs. Essentially, dabs is to weed, what crack is to cocaine. Most kids and parents have no idea at all about this. Most parents I have met had no idea what dabs, butter, K2, wax and concentrate even were.

What I am hearing from young people is the belief that smoking dabs with a vapor cig or E cig is that they think it's considerably less harmful than smoking regular weed thru a pipe. They believe this is a clean drug. How they were able to incorporate that thinking is beyond me. Many of these kids use butane torches to smoke with or the lighters filled with butane vapor. The kids definitely get that it is potent, but appear to have no awareness that it's harmful and that the butane impacts their brain chemistry in big ways. A couple of kids used dabs as a detoxing tool from heroin, due to its potency. The dabs helped make the withdrawal process a little better. It is called dabs, because all it takes is a dab of it to get wasted. A dab will do the job. Despite the potency of dabs, you can obtain dab wax easily and cheaply over the net including on sites like E bay and Amazon, where they both sell the wax needed to extract weed into dabs. The butane is also easy to get over the net because it is basically lighter fluid.

Some of the conversations I have had with kids using and making dabs is very revealing. Several of the kids I interviewed dislike dabs because it can incapacitate them leaving them unable to do anything while high. These kids report the lack of desire to have sex when on dabs and an inability to drive or even perform other daily activities. One kid compared his high on dabs to that of being on ketamine, a cat tranquilizer. A very sweet young 18 year old came to the institute, driven by her mom, and told me right away that she had just smoked some very potent wax in a vapor cig and that I should not expect much work to go on today. I asked her why she decided to come and if she could tell me what she was experiencing at that moment:

> "I am so wasted. It's really too much, like I can't do anything. Just coming up your stairs was hard. I can hardly feel my body or anything. It's just too intense. Weed is mellower and you can at least get stuff done, here you're just wasted. But, I use it a lot because regular weed is just not doing it for me anymore. I need to smoke all day long and can't sleep without smoking, so I am trying more dabs to keep that high."

I sent her home to go to sleep and met with her parents the next day. I know this young lady is not alone in her experience. Young people are getting medical weed from the west and using it to make this new, highly concentrated form of THC. It is everywhere, available for anyone who wants it.

There is a great web site I like called "The Fix." It is a great resource guide to all things related to addiction and recovery. It contains information on rehabilitation centers and sober living. It includes reader's forums where anyone can ask questions about using or recovery. "The

Fix" is a great tool for young people who often use the net for every-thing and prefer to communicate anonymously. I recently logged on to the site to find a post called, "Is dabbing the Crack of Pot?" The post clearly states that dabs can be harmful and that the butane is also dangerous.

My initial intention in this chapter was to list the strains and po-tency of each of the above mentioned substances. I have decided not to do that as the information is readily available on the web. I will pro-vide, however, a snap shot of what information is out there.

- The magazine *High Times* came out with their top pick of the year. It was a toss-up between "Girl Scout Cookies" and "PurpleUrkel." Another popular product was "The Golden Goat," a sweet and sour hybrid that has a reputation around how bad it smells. "Train Wreck" was also very popular.

- The web site "Medical Marijuana Strains" reviews a lot of strains of weed. They were big proponents of "Blue Dream." "Blue Dream" was claimed to be 80% Sativa. There is some literature indicating that Sativa can be helpful for depression, bipolar disorder, migraines, stress, and anxiety.

- We came cross a strain called "Purple Dragon" claiming to give you energy and increase motivation. This product came in 25% THC. "Lemon Diesel" came in at 14% THC while "Bruce Banner #3" (I guess there were others, 1, 2?) came in saying they are the best at 28.35%!

- A lab called Cann Labs claims to be the leader in the industry for innovative cannabis testing.

- "Learn Growing" is a web site that works with anyone wishing to grow and sets up seed deliveries.

- Even the UN has a site!! "United Nations on Drugs and Crime." They put out something called "The World Drug Report."
- The University of Washington has a decent site about potency. This site informed its readers that true bud lies at the very top of plants. But, most true pot smokers already know that.
- One article (Addiction Journal, vol 103, issue 7) provided statistics on the increasing amount of THC in marijuana throughout the years. In the 1960's THC levels were 7-12%, 1970's 10-12%, with a huge jump in 2008 to 15%. This percentage keeps going up.

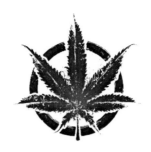

WHAT'S IN THE BUD?
THE UNKNOWNS AND BUD

If you are smoking a lot of weed you are not going to like this chapter. Please do not skip it. Read it because it has information that you need to know! For a young person who has found their way to this book, please understand that the intention is not to bring fear or any kind of judgment. If you are a parent of a young person who is frequently using weed, you need to know this information so you can parent effectively and have a firm grasp on how high the possibility is that your kid is ingesting a very toxic product.

We have two growing industries, legal and illegal. You would assume that most medical weed grown is safe and toxin free. You would also assume that most illegal weed grown, perhaps by cartels or gangs, may not be as safe. This chapter will present the facts and information regarding both. So what is in the cannabis plant (aka: bud)? Cannabinoids are groups of chemical compounds found in the cannabis plant. They affect both the body and mind through their interaction with cannabinoid receptors found throughout the immune, digestive, reproductive, central, and peripheral nervous systems of humans as well as animals. The activation of cannabinoids is what leads to the medicinal effects of bud.

Tetahydrocannabinol (THC) is the most well-known cannabinoid and the one responsible for causing the sensation of being "high." The psychotropic nature of this chemical can heighten the senses making music seem more intense and colors more magnified. THC also has broncho-dilating, anti-asthma effects. It is also an analgesic (pain reducer), it can sharpen the mind, induce anxiety if taken in large doses, and can stimulate appetite. Tetahydrocannabivarine (THCV) greatly enhances THC, inducing stronger buzzed highs, giving impact and power to the strain. Its effects are quick to come on and fade just as quickly. THCV is essentially THC's antagonist diminishing appetite. It is also pain reducing and euphoria inducing. Cannabidiol (CBD) works an opposite effect from THC reducing the psychoactive effect of THC, lessening the euphoric feelings felt by slowing down the metabolism of THC within the liver resulting in a prolonged effect of the THC. Users will often feel the type of cannabinoid in their muscles. It is a sedative and analgesic. CBD also contain an anti-spasmatic component which helps to relax muscle spasms. Unlike THC and THCV, CBD is not psychoactive. Cannabigerol (CBN) is somewhat of a psychotropic with a very strong pain killing effect. It is most useful with patients who have headaches, arthritis, and difficulty sleeping and is said to be three times as effective as aspirin for pain relief. Large concentrated doses of CBN can cause some level of disorientation. Cannabigerol (CBG) has a highly narcotic effect but is not addictive. I can help with sleep, killing germs (as it possesses microbial properties), and lowers the pressure inside the eyes, thus good for glaucoma patients. Finally, Cannabichromeen (CBC) can amplify the effects of THC producing a much more intense feeling of euphoria. Like all the cannabinoids, it has a sedative effect and is known to help relieve pain.

Now that we know what is in the weed the next question is, "Is weed an addicting substance?" According to a 20 year study by Professor Wayne Hall from Kings College in London, weed is not only massively addicting it is also harmful to an individual's mental and physical health. Professor Hall's study found that 15% of young people who smoke weed regularly are dependent on it and have difficulty quitting. In fact, his study indicates that it is harder to get people who are addicted to weed off of it than it is to get addicts off heroin. Withdrawal from marijuana includes anxiety, insomnia, loss of appetite, and depression. More than half of those that do quit return to use within six months. The recovery rate for weed is similar to that of alcohol and is very low, approximately 20%.

During the early 1980s the US Government executed a plan to destroy Marijuana crops in this country. Florida was the first state to have a substance known as paraquat sprayed on the bud plants. Paraquat is a toxic chemical that is widely used as an herbicide (plant killer), primarily for weed and grass control (Center for Disease Control). The Florida Department of Law Enforcement sprayed the paraquat on an 80 acre field in the Florida panhandle. When this event took place, an organization called the National Organization for the reform of the marijuana laws fought in court to block paraquat spraying, contending that any paraquat loaded weed would find its way to consumers and into the marketplace and that it would definitely pose a health hazard to the consumer. The paraquat remaining on the sprayed weed would have huge impacts on the user's health and many unknown factors surrounding the levels of toxicity. Apparently the Drug Enforcement Agency (DEA) did not fully understand the potential harmful effects of the chemical paraquat. Currently paraquat can be used only by people who are licensed applicators. Although use of the chemical is now regulated, at one time it was one of the most powerful weed killers known, while its fall out on the health of human consumption was unknown and also denied by the US government for some time. The US Environmental Protection Agency classifies paraquat as "restricted use." However, paraquat from outside the United States may not have these safeguards added (Center for Disease Control).

For several years, paraquat was used to spray weed farms in Kentucky and Georgia. The powerful chemical in it is Dimethyl-4, a viologen that is deadly. It can kill green plant tissue on contact and is highly toxic and not meant for human consumption. It has also been linked to the development of Parkinson's illness. Should a human smoke weed with any paraquat on it, as many did in the 1980s, they would come down with symptoms of major organ failures, such as liver, lungs, heart, and kidneys. Within days and weeks of ingestion they became deadly ill.

Also in the 1980s the Mexican Government, with the USA approving to support the war on drugs, began to use paraquat to combat the increasing number of illegal weed growing farms. Several fields were sprayed in the state of Chihuahuahur resulting in the killing of a child and causing over three hundred people in the town to become violently ill. These people had nothing to do with the growing and farming of weed, but were in close physical proximity to many fields, thus it was assumed they did, but no proof was ever verified. The Mexican town of Chorow was also sprayed. How a town could be misplaced for a weed field, I don't truly understand. Panic unfolded as many lost vision, airways and mucous membranes were affected. Of course the Mexican government denied any claims that they harmed anyone, except a few chickens and cows.

In 1984 the toxic chemical was banned and in 1985 the Governor of those towns was still claiming that paraquat was not harmful. The everlasting war on drugs has many unknowns in it, but it certainly has not been successful if we went from spraying highly toxic chemicals on illegal plants to using highly toxic chemicals on legal plants now.

An interesting side note to this story is "The Case of the Frozen Addicts" which was told in detail in the book written by Langston and Palfreman (2014) called just that. In certain areas of the country many heroin addicts came down with Parkinson like symptoms and some with the actual disease. It turned out that criminal chemists were making batches of a synthetic form of heroin to sell for profit and to evade the law as they could not be arrested for a substance not yet known and classified by the DEA. These chemists developed a drug that was completely unknown, which was often referred to as "Super Demoral." The chemicals used in the processing of the super D was methyl 4 and MPTP (both killed nerve cells and were also in paraquat). Heroin addicts who became sick and started showing up in emergency rooms in Baltimore and Philadelphia city hospitals with Parkinson like symptoms provided a huge clue and link between pesticides and illnesses like Parkinson's. The super D was as strong as an opiate like substance. The result was a large mass of individuals seeking out the substance out on the streets as is often the case when any powerful bag of dope gets word of mouth around being really good. Addicts are always searching for the most powerful bag and not really paying much attention to the fall out the bag may bring. Such is the nature of late stage addiction.

These designer chemical bags of heroin have surfaced many times over the years, some containing the powerful drug fentanyl in them as well. During the making of these designer drugs molecules can shift under heat and other unknowns creating a powerful high. The result is a deadly unknown chemical reaction in the brain around the dopamine receptor site instead of the endorphin receptor site where most opiates often go. This link from "The Frozen Addicts" makes it clear that MPTP and MPPP are extremely toxic to humans predominately impacting the dopamine receptor sites. There is a rare brain chemistry event existing in approximately 15% of users called the dopoengineric brain syndrome, where all substances used end up going to the dopamine receptor site areas. Here both the endorphin and dopamine sites are both stimulated.

Science is becoming increasingly concerned about all of the unknowns of substance use, particularly marijuana. As noted above, there are so many factors involved and so little known about how certain chemicals are impacting the brain. We are just breaching the surface when looking at the impact of pesticides in the soil of marijuana crops as well as the chemical reactions that occur when heating the paraphernalia used to smoke marijuana. The unknowns of laced weed with chemicals such as K2 and spice as well as homemade dabs with hot butane pipes containing copper create a very dangerous situation for brain chemistry. Street dealers simply change a few ingredients and a new unknown is sold in corner groceries around the Bronx, Harlem, and many other inner city areas. Do we truly have any clue as to the synergistic effect of all these substances entering the brain and often remaining there?

Some young people are buying synthetic weed like products over the internet. There is a site called synthetic M. alternatives selling all types of legal substances like sonic boom. Sonic boom is one of the newer strains of a reproduction of THC like chemicals that is very strong. So strong that some will prefer it to normal weed. Yet another site, Grassity.com you will find plenty of information about lacing and a recommendation to lace using DXM or Dextromethorphan. A big concern here is that most parents are completely unaware of the many web sites that sell illegal products that mirror weed, all chemical concoctions, with completely unknown impacts. This highly popular site, "The Silk Road," developed a skillful method of using Bit Coins, an underground economy, to purchase products. Recently the owner of "The Silk Road," after having made over forty million dollars, was sentenced to life in jail. "The Silk Road" was quickly replaced by another site, "Agora," which was up and running using the same bit coins. When they get shut down another site will come up. Word is spread by mouth. Kids tell other kids and these sites flourish. Many kids in the suburbs have access to their parents' credit cards or have their own debit cards to purchase illegal substances online. While the inner city kids are buying synthetic cocktails off of the street. These cocktails are constantly changing with completely unknown ingredients, giving a powerful high where one is left with bad headaches for days. My concern is who is going to take responsibility for these young people and their wellbeing? How can we expect parents to know about all these things?

Another unknown is how much chronic weed use changes the individual's belief systems and values. Can chronic use cause a shift from an intact value system to a skewed value system deviating from the individual's original views? As our culture moves towards legalizing weed, individuals have been given the green light to keep moving forward with their use. The fear of arrest and failure to get into college are no longer pressing concerns. I will not spend much time on values and belief systems as these are very individualized. Instead I will stick to the facts. We know that severe levels of toxins are reaching and affecting the brain, thus impacting thousands of young lives on a worldwide level. For all the unknowns around marijuana use there is substantial research around the adverse side effects of use. Dr. Nora Volkow's research found that the rise of marijuana use in young people brings health, social, and academic risks. She found that early weed use in life can interfere with crucial social and developmental milestones and can impair cognitive development (The New England Journal of Medicine, 2014).

The concept of medical weed is neither good nor bad. One can grow and consume a clean product and one can grow and consume a contaminated product. However, the concept that a sick person, who uses weed for health benefits could be consuming a toxic product is just unacceptable. It is tragic and a completely another unknown. A good question is why are there not more studies from those making huge profits from both legal and medical weed. I believe that the states, who imposed a 30% tax rate, can put some of that money into reducing any contamination levels in medical and legal weed.

A farm like the Stanley's out in Colorado spent time and money extracting the CBD from the THC and grew the well-known Charlotte's Web strain for children with epilepsy. They are proof that one can grow a clean product and help with medical problems while making a good profit and creating harmony in life alleviating suffering for many. That a country like Israel can be twenty years ahead of us in research and has managed to also make a clean product with no toxicity, create funding for research, and have complete control over the bud is amazing and perhaps a model that we in the USA need to look at closer and follow.

As in the beginning of this book where weed is concerned it is not a good or bad thing. Some are hurt and some are helped by it. Yet it is clear to me that as far as the impact on our young people, most are having harmful fall out if they are using it addictively. As we move headstrong into legalization and more medical use all of the factors raised in this book need to be looked at and addressed. Contamination must be reduced as a public health risk. Butane and copper tanks should not be as readily available on the internet for kids of all ages to purchase. We don't want a generation of zombies. A generation of young people whose brains are hijacked from so many unknowns. Instead, we wish for our youth to have a healthy, productive, and happy life. To have the same chances we were given and to succeed at things they want to create for themselves. We want all kids, from all walks of life, suburbs and inner-city, to realize their dreams and to make full use of a healthy growing and evolving brain. Let those that can afford to, and have the facilities, create more research around all the topics here in true bud. Such huge amounts of profits that are now being made in the Green Rush can be diverted so some of it goes into limiting the fall out for those that end up smoking and using chronically. Our hope is that all the unknowns will become knowns, and all dreams will become reality.

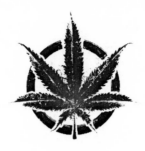

STORIES FROM BIRD

Comments from JA:

I am a young man, 21 years of age, who has been around BIRD since I was 14 years old. I feel safe at bird and was asked by Scott to write something up around dabs for his book. I have made dabs that can be a clean product, but most dabs are not. It is much more time consuming to make it pure and clean. This is what I am seeing mostly with the dabs that are around most kids today. Modern methods used to extract THC and cannoiboids include alcohol, butane, CO_2, chloroform, and other solvents. The outcome is honey bells, an oil like substance. Although the purity is greater than regular weed or hashish, there is definitely the risk of injecting toxicity. The concentrated dabs, I see around with friends, is often polluted and is making them total stoners for real. Solvents were not meant to be ingested and are NOT good for anyone. Do most kids truly care about this? I have found that they do not. Most dabs mess with both your physical and even more so your mental health. Butane sucks and is really bad for you and even though I made a formula of dabs without it, you still needed to smoke it with a butane tank. I have learned through Scotts work here at BIRD that this is very detrimental.

A Story from CV:

When I was younger I lived in a small village called Lake Placed. Although we eventually moved to a different residence, my family kept our beautiful rustic Adirondack home on the lake. It would always be a place for us to return to. The view of the lake and the mountains were serene and peaceful Lake Placid was a place where I brought friends to enjoy the serenity I knew it had to offer. We spent a lot of our summers there due to my entire family's love for the place. It was the end of August 2013, and my sophomore year of high school was approaching. The year before I was struggling with myself. My mind was forcing my body into starvation mode. I was a full blown anorexic that couldn't be stopped. My family and friend feared my life was at risk so they decided treatment was the only option for me.

It was right around Christmas, three weeks before I had to leave for a recovery center in Denver, which I drank myself wasted for the first time. I was 13 years old and having an empty stomach all of the time made it and easy task. It was the first time was free of my own mind. At that moment I knew being in an altered state was the only way for me. At the end of January, I was sent away, leaving my brooding school in Kent, CT, never to go back. I was discharged from treatment in April. Over the course of that summer I would get drunk quite often. I drank more and more as the summer went on. At the end of the summer in Lake Placid, I went out with my friend Lauren. We were wandering the one street town trying to decide what to do with our open night. I remember that night clear as day. Lauren know I never smoked weed before so she asked, "Do you want to smoke some bud?" A smile lit up my face and curiosity flickered in my still wide eyes. We walked only a few minutes in the crisp night air and ended up at a couple run down looking houses. We walked into the one on the left after she called up to the guy whom the house belonged to. We took off our shoes and walked up the creaky stair case. We sat down at a wooden table and she pulled out a bowl and a rather decent amount of weed, probably a little over a quarter. Lauren picked the bud off the stems and the aroma that filled the air aroused my senses. I had never smelled anything so satisfying. As soon as she packed a fat bowl she taught me how to take a hit. By the third hit I was a pro and felt the impact. The world felt like it was sliding from right beneath me. Everything was spinning. The only kind of spinning you get from being high. It is not the dizzy kind of spinning. After experiencing the high for a bit and enjoying myself a little too much we started drinking. I remember thinking to myself that weed was possibly better than booze. I didn't have a care in the world. I tried my first cigarette that night and liked the harsh flavors of the Marlboro red resting between my index and middle finger. I went home in a better mood than I had ever felt. My family didn't even care about the smell of booze, weed, and cigarettes. They didn't think anything of it. They were just relieved to see me happy. The next day I smoked wee again. This time we smoked in the woods. I remember seeing the leaves and being sure that they were dancing before me. I remember laughing a lot with my friend as we headed into town to satisfy our munchies. I was so nervous going into the bagel shop because the owner was good friends with my mom and my eyes were red and low.

As the summer had ended and I had to attend a new school, I was determined to become friends with the stoners. I had begun a different lifestyle. Finding people who liked smoking just as much as I did ended up being a very easy task. With my new friends, I managed to smoke almost every day and I had only started about a month before. For the first time in my academic career, my grades were slipping. I just didn't care anymore. The most important thing was getting stoned. I skipped class to go smoke with my friends. I would leave school in the middle of the day and go on a different adventure always revolving around weed. Would go with my friend, Abigail, and we would have to figure out ways to get money, find a dealer that wasn't dry, find a way to get a piece, etc. Most of the times the money would come from my parents. I would tell them I needed money for lunch or I owed a friend. A lot of the time my friend and I ended up using tin foil or aluminum cans because we just didn't care and all of our money would be gone at that point. This was just the beginning of my relationship with weed. Eventually I ended up getting caught by my parents and the school. This happened on more than one occasion.

In October 2013 I dropped acid for the first time. My mom found out because of my careless mistake of leaving Facebook open on her iPad. I remember the day my mom, bRosser and sister confronted me. My bRosser had always meant the world to me as did I to him. I was closer to him than anyone else particularly during this time when my relationship with my mom was becoming rockier by the day. I loved drugs more than anything in the world. I spat cruelly at my family. For the first time in my entire life I saw my bRossers eyes fill up with hot tears as I told them that drugs would always come before them and I didn't care what it took to get my hands on them. I was on a toll. I couldn't stop myself. The ugly truth was coming out in front of the people that should have been the last to hear it. They saw me ruining my life right before their eyes again. The truth was I was sick of rules. I was sick of people trying to help me by telling me what to do and how to live my life. Weed made me feel independent. It was my escape.

Looking back at this incident now I feel that all of my humanity and warmth had vanished. I still didn't stop. If anything things started heating up with my drug use. I had already gone through my first few bowls, my mother always finding them and confiscating them. In November, I went to school with a bowl in my bag along with only a gram of bud. At this point my now blue-green ombre hair and excessive absences in class gave the school enough reason to search my bag. It wasn't a great day. I rebelled against all of them because weed gave me the confidence to stand up for what I felt was "right." This wasn't the first time the school had caught me. However, this time they weren't as forgiving, suspending me for two weeks and calling the New Castle police. I was lucky that I was still 15 because I got put on a PINS instead of going to jail. I remember them telling me that if I were 16, which was only two months away, I would be in jail. PINS stands for Person In Need of Supervision. As a result of the PINS I was subjected to mandatory drug testing. In addition it did not allow me to leave the state and it wasn't prohibiting me from getting my permit on my 16th birthday.

Once a week, on Tuesdays, I would have to drive 20 minutes in the car with my mom to go get drug tested by a parole officer. She would come into the bathroom with me and watch me pee pitifully in the cup. I was always nervous knowing I wouldn't pass. I couldn't spend more than two days sober. It didn't take me long to realize the only thing she was testing me for was THC. That's when I discovered coke and pills. I had spent almost three weeks without THC entering my system when I went to get tested again. I was so proud and was confident I was going to pass the drug test. My parole officer didn't like me very much. She was a hardened, up tight woman, probably in her late twenties. She didn't seem to like anything to be honest. Yeah, she was one of those. I technically passed the test but she was skeptical. I screwed around with the last test I took, which she knew of course, so she wasn't sure if she believed the results this time around. With a little help from cocaine, that was the first and last drug test I would pass.

It was very apparent that the drug testing stressed my poor helpless mother out. She always looked so out of place there. It was obvious she was a lady with money and class that didn't belong there. She enjoyed pointing that out to me each time we went to the court house. I began smoking weed again and started to get attached to sniffing that powder a little too much. In the beginning of January 2014, I had another bag search. The school knew that I was high that day, which I was, but at this point I was a pro at passing their tests. When I got high, I wasn't out of control anymore. I could control my words and actions. I acted almost completely normal because it had become my new normal. The nurse told the principals that I passed the test and I was sober. I thought I was free to leave because I was 100% sure my bag was all clear. Turned out I was wrong. I didn't realize I had a dollar bill in my bag. It wasn't a normal bill. It was ripped in half, rolled up, with powder residue on it. I tried talking my way around it, telling them it was my medication and not coke. I was suspended for only one day. I went home after a meeting with the Principal and two assistant principals and the car ride with my mom wasn't a pleasant one. For the first time she had told me I was a disappointment. I had failed as her daughter. "You're a fucking bitch!" I scowled at her and with that she hit me three times which was something I used to get a lot of as a child but not recently. Her and my father were Italian born and raised. It wasn't abuse it was custom and discipline. For the first time, I clenched my fists and wanted to hit her back so badly. My anger had seemed to increase as the year went on. It was hard for me to control it without a substance. I was prepared to leap out of the moving car when she grabbed me tightly by my hair and yanked me back in before I was about to jump.

Of course I still didn't stop using after this. Instead I was experimenting with coke, molly, acid, salvia and pills. I was smoking cigarettes daily which my parents accepted after my doctor convinced them that it's okay that I smoked if it helped me not use. I played that card for a while. Eventually towards the end of January weed and coke were my best friends and I wasn't planning on letting them go anytime soon. I was using both daily, coke multiple times a day. Now it was Tuesday and it was about that time for me to go to PINS. I had a marijuana brownie before because I couldn't go in there and deal with the anxiety of that place remotely sober. The only positive thing that came out of PINS was meeting my current therapist, Scott Gillet. I had never had a therapist so laid back and easy to talk to. I liked him instantly. Talking to him was like talking to a friend filled with wisdom that only comes with age and experience. He didn't believe in PINS and tried to get me out of there but sadly even he didn't have the power over the law. Those days I was so worried about hiding the coke from my mom that I kept it on my person at all times and never in bags. I was so out of it that day that I forgot that the coke was still on me when I entered the court house. I walked in and the cop at the metal detector told me to empty my pockets and when I did, I felt a pill bottle. I knew it was my coke. Of course they saw it. Thankfully the other baggie I had was in my bra. That may sound strange but anyone who uses knows that that is one of the safest places to put an illegal substance. I told them the same thing I told my school. The coke was my medication that I crushed up. At the time I had a prescription for Zoloft, so I was lucky because that made it more believable. If it weren't for my mother, my ass would've been hauled to jail or boot camp at that very moment. The cops asked her if she wanted them to test it or flush it down the toilet.

I might as well have stopped before going through the metal detectors and told the cops to give me a second and let me finish my blunt.

My friends and family believed that the only reason I did that was because I wanted help. This wasn't true. If I wanted help I wouldn't ask for it from the police! I had no choice but rehad in Tucson, Arizona for three months. I lied and manipulated those people so much convincing them I was never going to use again and I felt like a completely different person. I knew the drill. If you didn't life all it lead you to was more treatment and I hated treatment. I was done! When I was finally let out in May 2014, I got drunk within the first week and picked up cigarettes again. I hadn't smoked weed in three months but to be honest, I was scared to. My parents were testing me when I got out of rehab. The only thing preventing me from smoking was the thought of leaving my life behind again and getting sent away for a longer period of time. I got drunk every couple of days though, trying to make sobriety work as much as I could. I went to NA meetings, saw my therapist, I started group therapy, the whole process. I went four months with no weed. Then one day, I was hanging out with my best friends, Tyler and Blake. They were ripping bong hits which was absolute torture for me. I loved bongs so much!! I had a beautiful one with mushrooms on the side of it and beautiful intricate patterns. When my mom found it last Christmas, she didn't smash it or throw it away. That relieved me because she gave it to someone she knew who would make good use out of it. Blake would provide me alcohol when they were smoking and I always had my cigarettes. I was starting to form a relationship with Tyler who helped me as mush as he could and was the greatest guy a girl could ask for. He treated me like I was a princess, but I was too lost and needed to figure myself out. I didn't see how he would drop everything for me. When I was hanging out with him and Blake at Blake's house he had to go get his haircut which only took an hour. Blake was the one person who shared the same amount of love for Mary Jane as I did. We spent a lot of time researching to see how many days before the test I could smoke. I finally caved in. I said "fuck it" and ripped that bong not 30 seconds after that. Four months without weed. Four months! It was euphoric and perfect. One I realized I wouldn't get sent back to treatment for smoking, the cycle started again. But this time it became even more intense than before rehab. I started smoking again in the summer of 2014 which made it easier to be stoned all day long.

Once my therapist and parents realized they couldn't stop me from smoking, they didn't even try. It started off with a bargain…keep it to the weekends. I tried to do this but it was never a success. Eventually they accepted it all together. (Author's note: This is her perception but it was distorted by bud. Both by myself, BIRD, her parents and another clinician involved never ceased to intervene on her. At the time of this writing she is clean and sober and very happy.) I couldn't' do without pot anymore. I smoked at least four times every single day. No matter where I was I could spot a dealer a mile away. No one was a better stoner. It's what I was best at. I could out smoke anyone. I had the coolest pieces, the best weed, and I provided the best hook ups to all of my stoner friends. Eventually the proud feeling I had when people would say they didn't know anyone who could smoke as much as me or when they would say I was such a stoner became almost hurtful.

As my junior year started I had a hook up for the best medical weed from the city and became very fond of dabs (or wax…whatever you want to call it). I had a dab pen and brought it with me everywhere. Dabs were for the go and the medical weed was kept at home with my blue skull bong. By junior year I changed my look to blonde hair, minimal makeup and "normal" teenage girl clothes. I had become a bigger pot head than ever before and hid it harder than ever. Since the school year started I cut back on drinking and upped the smoking. At this point I wasn't even getting high anymore. My tolerance was beyond high. It takes at least a couple of bowls to myself to get the buzz that I'm so accustomed to. Getting high wasn't exciting anymore. I still felt the need to do it though. I don't know if you can be addicted to marijuana but I was spending almost $400 a week on pot by October of 2014. I would smoke other people up but for the most part it was all mine. When it came to weed, passion and interest strikes up in me. I haven't felt a strong passion towards anything since before my eating disorder. Pot was the first thing I had felt excited about in a long time. It enhances all my senses. I study each strain carefully by smelling each one and appreciating the pungent aroma. I examine the detailed perfection of each nug, the shade of green it is, whether it's purple or has orange hairs. I had my preferences, specifically Buzz and Mr. Nice Guy. Each strain almost 25% THC. You can't get much better than that. Pot makes me feel passion for myself and only myself. It's selfish in that it won't let me love anything the same way I love it. I can't find joy in anything unless I'm high. I can't find the spark in anyone unless I'm high. If I feel my mind is too worn out and I'm too burnt out, something inside me pushes me towards the lighter, the grinder, a piece, and my weed. If I know I've had enough for one day or shouldn't have it at times, I can't help myself.

My friend Lauren always used to tell me, "Whenever someone mentions the word weed your brain turns to mush." She reminded me of what it did to me, how when it came to getting my weed I would do anything to have possession of it. I would easily ruin relationship s for pot. I would let my future go up into flames for pot. I would lose all self-respect for pot. But I never wanted to admit that. I never could because of fear of having to let go for the living in constant fear and anxiety of running out and not being able to get more. Sleeping, eating, homework, family events, social gatherings are all foreign to me unless stoned. It's not life threatening like the Anorexia or the coke, but it's lonely, empty, and meaningless. It makes me feel all these things.

I have become too attached too quickly and now I don't know how I will ever let go. Every time I leave my home town for what's supposed to be a relaxing vacation or a rare experience I get struck by fear and become a jumble of nerves knowing that I have to step out of my comfort zone and out of my way to look for pot in a completely foreign place. In the past these actions have lead me to questionable situations with sketchy people. During the summer of 2014, I was in Vermont for about a week or so with my sister and mother. My mother was thinking I would be taking a break from smoking. My sister is a serious horseback rider so I decided I would join her and watch her compete. The first day at the horse show I was determined to find my pot. I saw a man who was a stabile hand who traveled around with the horse shoes. Something in me told me he smokes and possible sells too. I caught him checking me out a few times before I made sure no one was around. I stomped on my cigarette and strutted toward him. He was probably in his late twenties, from Mexica, and it was a piece of cake. What I asked him if he know who sold he said that he was the guy. He gave me a free sample that day due to his strong attraction for me. As a girl it is easier to find bud than people think. The real pick up lead me to a hotel room full of men I didn't know asking me to stay and smoke with them. Not wanting to seem too concerned I took a couple of hits, grabbed my pot and made my way out. Not looking back. At 16 years old I went into a room full of Mexican drug dealers smoking and drinking for no more than 2 grams. I was desperate because I had gone almost 48 hours without smoking. For me it was unthinkable and not right. I had become too attached, too quickly, and I didn't know how to let go.

"Scott, I think I'm becoming retarded." That was how I ended my therapy session earlier this week, November 25, 2014. The last few days have been spent with my father in Lenox, Massachusetts at a Kripalu

Yoga center where you're supposed to relax and for me take a break. I haven't smoked in almost three days. This is the longest I have gone in almost five months. Cravings are constant and thorough. They never seem to diminish or lack detail. Each craving is joined by a vivid image of me braking up the weed, placing it into my silver grinder while turning it in each direction until it's perfectly ground. Then I pack a nice bowl or pack my bong and take the first hit of a fresh bowl. Savoring the familiar taste of the weed smoke. My whole body and mind ache for it. Everything white looks like a joint, certain smells trick my mind into thinking its pot. It's cruel that it does this to me and sometimes I hate it. I hate how much I love it. I'm lost without it but I'm also lost when I have it. My dad made me admit that even though most of it is bad, I'm not as physically and mentally drained. Sobriety is also letting me think more clearly and I'm able to remember things that were said to me five minutes ago. The down side is I don't have any motivation to do things that usually give me joy. I don't want to listen to music, it makes me think of getting high and how much better music is when you're blazed. I don't get excited to eat and neither does my stomach because it's better when you're high. Everything's better when you are high. Weed has made it so that I can't enjoy the things I used to unless I have it by my side. It's harder to let go of than my other addictions because it's better. It's not as miserable as the other stuff. The euphoric high has made it hard for me to see the negatives. The artificial happiness hides the undesirable bleakness.

One day later....I grabbed my two small bags from the car, speed walked to my room and plopped them on the wooden floor with confusing patterns on them. I helped unload the rest of the luggage from the yoga retreat and dropped it all on my kitchen. After that I practically went into a run knowing that it was finally time to get stoned. On my mini voyage I slipped on the confusing wooden floor plan, but that didn't stop this white girl. I got right back up and found my bong, bowl, gas mask, and dab pen just sitting there waiting for me to use them. I packed my dab pen within ten minutes of being home. I packed it four times before feeling settled. My parents believing it was brownies instead of the sour diesel crumble. My mother approved of the edibles believing they were better for you than smoking. The smoking concerned her. Lung Cancer and any sort of cancer runs in my family. From my grandparents, to my aunts and uncles, and both of my parents. Almost seven years ago my mom was diagnosed with Colon Cancer. Right around Christmas. They caught it early enough that she ended up being oaky after surgery. We were living in Brazil at the time. My dad's business is there so because of that we lived there for a couple of years testing the waters. Turns out the waters weren't so enjoyable to swim in. One year later, my dad was diagnosed with lung cancer. He never smoke cigarettes, it's all because of his unfortunate genetics. He had a 50% chance of or maybe even a 75% chance of making it. He eats health and exercises daily, so his "baby like" lungs worked to his benefit. Thankfully both of my parent are doing well now. However, my habit of smoking tobacco sticky and puffing ganja distresses them.

I'm convinced it's my genes. When I got home from that retreat I couldn't stop myself. I ripped from the bong, shared a joint, had some dabs, took some bong hits, and dabs again. I can usually control the munchies but this time I went all out. Five days without weed made me smoke weed until I passed out. When I finally had some it felt like I hadn't smoked in months. I questioned myself, "Was it really only five days without weed?" This is when I realized something….I am addicted to marijuana.

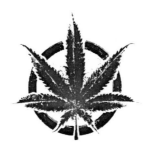

The Interview with Jeff
A Previous Member of the
W9 Gangsters

It is a hot July night and I am walking down 125th street. I can hear and see the trains coming and going out of the Harlem station. I used to take that train to work when I had an office in NYC, but tonight I drove down and walked because I had some time to kill. I spent some time in Harlem as a teen so I knew my way around. In 1969 you found very few white folks walking around, especially at night, but time has changed and transformed Harlem in many ways. Harlem now consists of some fine restaurants, and just about every sneaker store you could desire with all the latest kicks. You can even spot Bill Clinton occasionally. There is also a lot of expensive and very upscale housing. Harlem looked very different in the late 60s and early 70s. I started to wonder where all the original dwellers went. Where are they living now?

I was never afraid back then and I am not tonight. I'm excited about this chance to sit down with someone willing to talk about themselves and their gang experience around weed. It had taken a while to get this sit down. A friend of mine who lives on 123rd street had arranged it and truthfully, I did not know what to expect or if it would even happen. I had doubt because several gang members who sold weed were not too willing to talk with me or expose themselves. I had several no shows and requests for large sums of cash for an interview. Interviews contingent upon buying the sellers products such as sour or diesel weed.

But I am here tonight waiting to meet with this former member of the W9 Gangster. I should be experiencing some level of fear but for some reason my brain only registers excitement!

When I get to 125th street and see my friend with someone, I know at least an interview will happen. I get introduced to Jeff. We say hello and walk over to one of the fast food places where I can buy him some dinner, which is all he requested in exchange for the interview. I ask Jeff why he has offered to participate in this interview to which he replies that he wants to help kids. He wants to see young teens avoid going down the same path he had. He proclaims that he wants to do some good in the world. And so we get into it.

Jeff is a tall, good looking, thin, black man who is 44 years old. He has survived a lot. I liked him right off. He was authentic and willing to tell me the truth about things. He was even willing to let me use his real name. Jeff was in a gang called the W9 Gangsters for six years until he was thrown out for stealing some of the gang's weed. "They could have killed me," he says, "but I was the young kid and the dumb one and some high up members saw me as a mascot, so I survived." Jeff also survived a stint in Attica in 1989. He smoked and sold a lot of weed but also had another drug problem. At some point the gang started to lace the weed with some powerful new chemical high that they were calling K2. Jeff loved K2 and could not just smoke regular weed, he needed weed with K2 in it or he smoked K2 alone. You should know that at one point K2 and spice, another chemical high that also gets laced with weed, was legal at the time. What was in it depended on how it was made and who made it. Jeff told me that his gang realized that the customer who bought the weed often liked the stronger laced product, even though they had no idea it was laced when bought. Some did not like it and would not buy laced weed. Never the less, Jeff became addicted to K2 and weed for a while. "The high," he tells me, "was such a rush. Felt like going up in a rocket and I loved it. It made my brain feel alive!" Jeff had sold a lot of weed while in the gang, predominately to kids between the ages of 13 to 20. Jeff became a selling machine for the gang. He was bringing in big cash, had a lot of customers and had what he would call "the life" until he got arrested for bulk possession and some other offenses ending up in Attica.

Spice and K2 are illegal now, but Jeff says it's all over the place. He estimated 40% of most weed sold around the inner city areas is laced with something. After a while talking, Jeff started to have some head problems. He began to have headaches and reported feeling like his brain was getting hijacked by bad thoughts and images that he couldn't stop. He attributed this to his use of laced weed and the use of K2. He feels that using weed so much and then moving into K2 has destroyed something in his head. Jeff really appears to disconnect so I spend some time explaining how the receptor sites work and some of the changes in brain chemistry that may have occurred. Jeff describes his feelings of remorse for selling weed to kids as young as 12 years old. He tells me he never would sell to a pregnant women. The brand he sold was called "Sour Sometimes." He informed me that if the gang had it available they would lace the weed with small amounts of PCP (another very powerful drug). I asked him if the kids they sold to really did not know what they were smoking or what may have been put into the bag. He sadly replies, "Yes" and tells me that he feels bad that there may be kids walking around with some of the same head problems that he struggles with on a regular basis.

Although Jeff has been thru a lot, he went back to smoking and using weed after he left the gang. He has tried to get periods of complete abstinence from this weed-K2 combo, but is very candid when he proclaims feelings of powerlessness when trying to quit. "I cannot step away from the rush of using and the rush that I also get from selling." Jeff will not sell to young kids anymore and no longer laces his product. He states, "I only sell a little. Just to make ends meet and get by." When in the gang, Jeff did not have to worry much about money. The gang was well organized and everyone knew their job and role and had surrendered being an individual for the good of the group and it ran along like a smooth machine. He prefers not to get into numbers around money and he starts telling a story to me, but then half way thru he can't remember how the story ended. He expresses how "sad" he feels, "like I totally wasted my life and would love to have a regular job and normal life."

We end up talking for several hours and I learn from Jeff that the gangs are becoming concerned about how the legalization of medical marijuana will impact their profit making ability when it comes to selling marijuana. The gangs feel they need to make their product more powerful in order to compete. Lacing is the most fiscally responsible way to do this. Weed is a huge income for them. It is their main money maker and they are now facing the possibilities of losing that as a source of income. After several hours of talking, we say goodnight. He tells me he will call me with the names of the chemicals that he used when he made K2. I doubted that was going to happen and it did not.

As I am driving home, I start to think about what I have been seeing in my office the last few years. I know more and more kids end up coming to treatment due to a bad lacing experience where they had to go to their parents because they were flipping out from smoking what they had thought was just weed. Just last week I saw a young man, 21 years old, who was at some type of weekend show with a lot of music and drugs. The kid came to therapy reporting feeling like he was crawling out of his skin and losing his mind. I drug tested him and we found ecstasy and cocaine in his saliva. I had asked him to be honest with me about what he used that weekend. He told me he only smoked and was blown away that additional substances were in his system without his knowing. He was reasonably upset to know he was ingesting these chemicals without his awareness or his consent.

After kids are seeing you for a while they tend to open up more around their use if they feel safe. I would have to say that just about every kid who came in for two, maybe three years had stories about lacing. They could tell right off the weed was laced by the smell and texture of it. Of course I have to ask, "Why did you smoke it if you thought it was lace?" I always get the same response, "I wanted to get high and it was all I had." Once again I return to my vision of trying to find out what is in these kids brains'. Are they okay? Has some chemical they used damaged something in their wiring and can it be healed? I am seeing a thread running through all of these chronic weed users with a lot of the same ways of using and the symptoms that linger even after they have stopped. I am now a certified Nutrient Therapist and know a lot more about the brain and weeds effect on it. I am thinking that just normal treatment, the way it is set up today, is never going to look at their brain chemistry and connect the problems they are having with what is happening in the brain.

One young female, a 17 year old kid I see, cannot sleep at all without weed. Another has no appetite without weed. Another cannot concentrate at all or focus without weed. I can go on. I feel good about going in and spending time with Jeff, but am also saddened by the thought that this great guy may never get his brain recovered in his life and there may be many others out there just like him. I am thinking that I used to assume once a kid stopped smoking all of the effects of smoking would slowly go away, but now I know that many will not naturally return to their normal levels of functioning and that we need to start to look at how to help them in other ways.

Prior to concluding this chapter I would like to share a little more information on K2 and Synthetic THC.

A note on K2:

The night that I was in Harlem Jeff informed me that K2 was around and available on many street corners. The reason why K2 became banned by the DEA is that so many teens were showing up in the ER with various physical and psychiatric symptoms. At first, nothing like this had been seen before. Poison Control had to be called in to find what these teens were ingesting. K2 is a synthetic marijuana invented by a Dr. Huffman at Clemson University in 1995. The doctor was studying cannabinoids and had come up with this synthetic version. Dr. Huffman found no medical benefits from it, but did find a lot of negative side effects. On the street there are versions of K2 called Spice, Blaze, and Genie, all with various chemicals in them. They often cause psychotic effects with hallucinations, extreme anxiety, and paranoid states both during and after use. Hospitals report rapid heartbeat, vomiting, reduced blood flow to the heart, and heavy metal residue.

Some of the chemicals that have been found in several of the synthetic weed include arecannanbicychohexanol, tryptamine, 4-methylbuphedrone, and dimethylhexyl. The synthetic weed binds to some of the same receptor sites in the brain that THC would bind to, only at a strength ten times greater. Thus a young person, out for a fun night with friends, who may decide to smoke some weed laced with K2 which may very well alter their life for years changing something in their fragile brain chemistry that can destroy their life for good. In a story on NBC news (Channel 6 in Florida) on May 31, 2012, there was a case of a teenager ending up at Jackson Memorial Hospital ER for treatment after smoking some laced weed called "Mango Cheese." The Doctor was concerned about brain damage because the receptor site involved here is directly related to schizophrenia.

Several months after conducting this interview I was flipping through the channels on TV and came across a show with a drug dealer making K2. He had poured acetone and other chemicals over potpourri or weed and packaged it in shiny bright packets that look like candy so younger kids will be attracted to them. Edibles are being made to be much more attractive to young kids. Although the marijuana edibles are meant for medical use, they are in everything from gummy bears, lollipops, jolly rancher type candies and also presented in bright wrappers that kids would be attracted to. The intention here is not to create fear in anyone. It is an illustrations of what has been unfolding in the world of teens who are using.

A note on Synthetic THC:

Synthetic THC is not new. Many hundreds of derivatives were developed in the 1950s and 1960s in academic and pharmaceutical circles. One such derivative was called Nantradol, which was available in a pill form for pain. Another was Levonantradol. There were clinical trials by Pfizer in the 1980s. At the time Pfizer was also working on something called CP-55-940. It was considered to be as powerful as morphine as an analgesic. It was never introduced to the public due to its psychoactive side effects. Interestingly what the company considered side effects are the very same sensations one is craving in using

THC. One derivative that did become a medicine was Nabilone. Later Marinol was available for the public and was very effective in treating HIV-AIDS. During the early part of my career I was an Oncology social worker and came across Marinol often. I was amazed by how well it worked on many symptoms like nausea, appetite, anxiety, and depression.

Both Dr. Wilson and Dr. Morris were kind enough to spend time with me on the phone discussing metal toxicity and mythelation issues. THC stays in the body and brain for a long time, much longer than any other substance. It is quite possible that it may also be a thick, oily substance in the brain and perhaps even sit on the receptor sites, lingering much longer than we ever knew or imagined. Another important factor is that weed stays in the fat soluble cells for much longer than we thought. Thus, in chronic weed use, traces of THC could leave a trail in the brain limiting the firing of transmitters in different brain regions. Add using these substances for long periods of time many times a day. This is a form of toxicity that has never truly been looked at close enough. In the brief amount of time this area has been studied you begin to see the brain as significantly impacted directly and indirectly.

As I began my research on this form of pollution caused by environmental factors, in this case substances used to lace weed and other synthetic THC products, I began to speak to a lot of doctors and treatment providers in the community gathering information about what they were seeing and hearing. I was deeply touched by the level of commitment within the community, especially the young people. They knew that something in their brains were not right. They were struggling and did not want to live that way anymore. Even, long after weed use had stopped, there were still many symptoms that troubled the kids and their families. Many had ideas about the study and the hope that with advanced science and research their lives would improve in such a way that they would experience less anxiety, depression, and apathy. They look forward to increased motivation and riding themselves of feeling stuck in time with no direction.

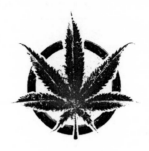

An Interview with an Organic Grower

JW is a very intelligent young man. At the age of 24 he heard the calling to "Go West Young Man." He had a hook up with a friend whose family had gone into the growing of good quality organic weed. JW had already tried many paths in his young life from being in a pretty good successful rock band to some school and some various marketing jobs. It seemed he had been around BIRD forever, but at some point had fallen in love, gone to AA, NA and got a few years clean and sober. He was loving his life and had worked really hard through some tough stuff to get to where he was. I always have a lot of respect for that and sometimes I am in awe around the miracle of where an individual was and where they brought themselves to. Yet, like most young people, JW was still finding his way in the world when an opportunity knocked on his door. He was invited to move out west to California and join a family farm business growing a good strain of organic weed for medical use.

There was much discussion about staying clean and sober and not testing or sampling the product, but this kid truly took his recovery seriously and was highly motivated to stay sober. He also had in his favor that fact that Alcohol was his drug of choice. His parents were naturally skeptical about his plan, but eventually all things were worked out and west he went. I chased JW down a few years later. He was doing fantastic! He wasn't using and he was going to meetings and keeping up with therapy sessions. His self-esteem was sky high and it was truly a beautiful thing to see.

The farm JW worked on was s a family operation in Sonoma County, California, a popular area for weed growth. JW was very willing to talk with me. Here are a few comments from the interview:

Scott - Would you know if Organic Fertilizers contain Nitrogen?

JW - The ones we use have Nitrogen, Phosphorus, and Potassium. Zinc is also important to growing weed. I will supply you with a list of our fertilizers and any pesticides, but we are organic and make a clean product for medical use.

Scott – Has your product even been tested for potency? If so, do you know how much the potency of your product is?

JW - I really don't and being I don't smoke anymore, I can't give you a more personal critique. We grow indoors and outdoors all year long. I know that the stuff grown indoors is more potent, but could not tell you why? The dispensaries sometimes test and there are labs around for potency telling you the exact amount of THC. But truthfully it is hard to keep track and there are so many strains, I just don't know.

Scott - What is the annual income for growers?

JW - For the farm workers it comes to $20 an hour. Work is seasonal, similar to working in vineyards. At the end of the summer there is always a big harvest, mostly mid-October and friends come to the farm and work along with us. It is a great time. We all connect, play music, go out and hang, and are like a big family. The family we work for sets the tone for the farm and they are good people. It is not uncommon to make $5,000 a month, but it's a lot of work. You have to be willing to work hard and the rest of the year your income could drop and fluctuate. Another big aspect is that we grow just for dispensaries, but most farms around divert the weed and grow for friends and for sale on the street all over the country. There is a law that will tell our farm how much our yield is allowed to be, but many farms grow as much as they want, and go way over the amount that the law states. For example in Sonoma County you are allowed to grow 30 plants per person and each person needs a medical marijuana card. Each plant produces 3-4 pounds, but it needs to be cleaned up and ends up less than that. Sold in California it would come to $150,000. It raises your income by growing indoors too. Of course, I'm not going to lie to you, a lot of weed makes its way to the streets and goes for much more, and that's where the real money is.

Scott - How much do you think you would get for a pound of your weed if sold on the street?

JW - Out here in California $1,300 to $2,300 wholesale. In New York $2,300 to $3,300. But hey, should I be telling you this stuff?

Scott - Listen, whatever you're ok with. I am not pressing you. Just tell me what you're comfortable with. Okay?

JW - Yeah, all good. I also wanted to tell you that this week, I worked like 50 hours.

Scott - How long is the growing season, planting to harvest?

JW – It goes from around June 1 to Oct 20.

Scott - What is the average age of the workers out here?

JW - 28-32

Scott - What keeps you from not being raided being lots of other farms are growing more than allowed?

JW - We obey the planting guidelines. Others may be growing hundreds of plants over the limit. There have been some raids recently. Police helicopters fly overhead and try to count plants, but there are lots of farms these days. Not just here in Calli, but Colorado and Washington State too. If you stay in the 90 plant range, you're OK.

Scott - Can you tell me how it works with where the products go? Do clients with cards come here to buy?

JW - Most go to dispensaries we have deals with. Clients with medical cards can buy right from the farm if they like. It's not like there is an official system in place yet. California is still working this stuff out.

Scott - How much money do you think farms diverting weed to the streets are making a year?

JW - Not sure if I want to go there. I trust you, but who knows where this information may end up? Look, it's the Wild West, the green rush. Money can be made and a lot of it. I dream about getting some land and having my own farm. That's why I am learning every aspect of the business. It's a good business that can help a lot of sick and ill folks. It's close to the earth and all natural. Some women from a farm nearby pray and meditate over their plants and send love to the plants and talk to the plants! Its weed, my man, it's going to be crazy.

I thanked him and commented on how far along he had come in his life and that he had learned to trust his instincts more in life and seemed more spiritual. JW replied, "Scott, sometimes at sunset I am out on my motorcycle riding in the hills and the bike is humming and my head is empty, like no mind and I am in harmony with everything in the world."

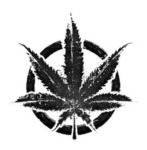

What's used in Organic Growing?

From my interview with JW, I was able to obtain a list of everything used to grow their organic product.

Here is what's used:

- Soil: 707 Formula by Aurora
- Nutrients added throughout the season: Pro Tekt by Dyna Gro and others from Greenhouse Megastore
- Other products used for growing:
    - o floralicious, koolbloom, diamond nector, floranova and roots exclurator

You may want to go back to the chapter titled, What's In the Bud? Here you will see what gangs are using to put in their weed and what farms that claim to be organic are putting in their planting process.

I want to make it clear that the goal here is not to teach or assist anyone in learning how to grow marijuana. True Bud is not about that. It is about understanding the concepts of contamination, the dangers and effects of pesticides, soil contamination and fungi that often grows in moist settings.

Washington State, where medical weed is also grown, has an extensive web site with strict guidelines around what products can and cannot be used in growing pot. It seems to me that every state needs to be moving in this direction. Without this transparency, it feels exactly the same as the bootleggers who made their home brews during the early part of the nineteenth century. When I spent time in India, I was amazed at what was being sold as an alcohol product. There were poor people who could never afford brand booze who were getting sick and many were going blind from alcohol poisoning. It was all they could afford to buy and they wanted to drink, but were abused by a system that did not provide the right controls and testing. Thousands of people die every day in India. Walking thru the slums of Mumbai, Bombay, I saw suffering and many drinking cheap homemade booze. Mothers were trying to feed their hungry children, while losing their men to poisoned booze. We cannot have the same things happening in the US because we are not investing the time and money into the regulation of marijuana.

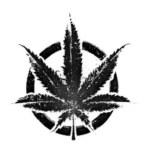

PESTICIDES IN CANNABIS

Let's start with a fantastic piece from the Journal of Toxicology (2013) entitled, "Determination of Pesticide Residues in Cannabis Smoke" where researchers found that pesticide toxicity is well documented. During the heating of pyrolysis, products from the plant interact with the pesticides forming more toxic materials. Exposure to phosphate pesticides thru inhalation caused the most rapid appearance of toxic symptoms and has even resulted in cases of death from respiratory failures. Those using medicinal cannabis may be more physiologically susceptible to negative impacts caused by these residues. In order to obtain a wide view in this very important study different pipes for smoking weed were used including a glass pipe and water pipes with both carbon filters and cotton filters. It was determined that the glass pipe had evidence of pesticides such as bifenthrin, diazinon, permethrin, and paclobutrazol.

A grower's crop is literally their income and their cash. The more the crop yields the more money a grower makes. Growers must use pesticides to fight off insects, mold, fungi, and other things that can destroy a crop. All of the chemicals enter into the soil. Weed is not a clean product and is rarely washed or hosed down before sold and distributed. To my recollection, I have not met many kids who washes the weed they use. According to one of the more popular websites on pesticides, bacteria, mold, and fungi can affect any plant crop, but the lack of regulatory restrictions in most states puts users of weed at an especially high risk (www.truthonpot.com). A recent Dutch study, which tested weed sold in 10 local coffee shops, found bacteria and fungi in all of the samples tested. One common bacteria was pseudomonas aevginosa. High levels of such bacteria can produce carcinogenic toxins called aflatoxins. In addition, the Harvard School of Public Health did a study that found the DDT pesticide will have effects on children and young people's neurodevelopment. They believe that ADHD and other learning disabilities that often develop in young people may come from what they are calling neurotoxicants. More and more exposure to these neurotoxicants is a direct result from smoking weed that may be toxic.

Another chemical used to grow weed is chlorpyrifos. Chlorpyrifos was banned in the USA in 2001 but is still used and easily accessible for any growers who want to use it. Studies have also linked this banned pesticide to ADHD and learning disabilities as well as to memory loss, the most widely known side effect of smoking. Despite banning the use of chlorpyrifos, its use remains very popular in the growing industry. Throughout my clinical experiences with teens who are chronic pot smokers, it is not uncommon that they need to be sent a text the day of their appointment or you may not see them. The kids text me constantly asking when is our appointment, what did you tell me to write, what was that assignment you gave me, what am I supposed to speak to my father about? And so on. There is no denying that something these children are doing is impacting their memory.

Dan Tomaski, who runs North Michigan's most comprehensive Medical Marijuana testing lab service, found that some weed contained mold and pesticides at levels more than 60 times those allowed. That's 60 times the proper amount! Store bought spinach tested lower. They go on to say that most consuming products like apples and vegetables are almost always washed before consumption and often washed again at home by the consumer. There is no system in place to wash or remove the toxins from weed (Mascagni, 2013). More recently Dr. Raber, a Ph.D. in Chemistry from the University of Southern California provided some important information. Dr. Raber runs the Medical Marijuana Testing Lab in Los Angeles. The Doctor says that up to 70% of pesticides found on marijuana buds can transfer to the smoke being inhaled, similar to injecting them into your bloodstream. He also noted that 35% of weed fails pesticide testing. He determined that these pesticides go directly up to the brain, unlike food, which goes thru the GI track.

Yet another study conducted by the Los Angeles city district attorney tested three samples of medical marijuana from California. All three samples had dangerously high levels of the insecticides Bifethrin. One of the samples was 1600 times higher than the normal and approved level. Now, think about this for a moment. This is medical marijuana, not street bud! This stuff is going to patients who are already ill. Some may have lung cancer and pre-existing respiratory problems. Does this mean that the medicine, weed in this case, is going to make them sicker? CNN recently covered big stories on their series, "High Profits." What these stories failed to report was that many plants are filled with toxins. Why would they fail to provide this information to the public? (Cashing in on the 'Green Rush', CNN, April 2015).

A website designed for growers of weed quoted a recent article from the Bay Citizen, "Pesticides not meant for use on common crops like weed are available in 'Grow' shops thru out the bay area (*www.**manicbotanix**. com)*." It is a bustling market in which toxic substances are sold over the counter in unmarked vials. This would mean that it would be virtually impossible for the FDA or DEA to be able to check every farm in the state of California. The bottom line is legal or illegal, growers want to produce a high yield that they can sell. They may have a license to sell, but they may not care or think they would ever be caught using banned or illegal products used for growing. Almost all pesticide use is illegal in growing weed, with the exception of specific approved ones. Illegal growers will do whatever they can to produce the most powerful THC content and the most amount of plants (*www.manicbotanix.com*).

I am no expert on pesticides or agriculture, so I went online to see what I could buy over the internet. I typed in the search bar, "need fertilizers and pesticides for pot." I was astonished at how many products were available just with a click of a button. I was also surprised to see that some of the products were labeled "highly toxic" such as diazinon, atrazine, chlorpirifos, pyrethrum, glyphosate. I could also get copper, which was made and used to control mold. I thought to myself, if high levels of copper were in the soil or plant would they end up in the consumer of whatever was grown? Let's hope someone who knows and understands these toxins can somehow get them out of the growers' hands. Many of the products used for growing weed are meant for lawns or tree spraying, not for human consumption. The research is showing that toxic chemicals are reaching the brain and having a direct impact on brain chemistry.

Although I have cited several studies on marijuana contamination, not much attention has been given to what's in the soil. We know that copper and mercury are in it, but there has been no attempt to see if those things end up in the plant. When conducting my research I came across several You Tube videos with growers discussing how to address the low levels of zinc in marijuana. Interestingly, almost all of the kids tested at BIRD for TMS had low or no zinc. Zinc is a major player in brain chemistry events and also in keeping copper levels balanced. I couldn't help but wonder if there is a connection between this problem growers experience and young people ending up low in zinc. The research tells us that weed lowers zinc. As a result, we at BIRD supplement all our users with zinc. It would make sense that whatever is in the soil may end up in the plant and that high levels of copper and mercury can impact the person ingesting the plant. We actually had one kid in our study have a level of mercury over 200 times the normal level.

When I conducted my interview with the organic grower, I was impressed by how much care the farm took in the use of chemicals. Products like koolbloom, diamond nector, and floralicious are used on the thriving farm crops. The Washington State Department of Agriculture (WSDA) has its own web site for weed growers. It clearly states that only pesticides and fertilizers approved by the state of Washington can be used. The site offers a link to WSDA products that must be used on any weed grown in the state of Washington. As the medical marijuana industry grows it will generate many millions of dollars. The farms and growers are all taxed if they are licensed to grow. Some states tax up to 30%, but is different in every state. A lot of resources will be needed to check all the farms to see if they are meeting regulatory guidelines. In Colorado, the green rush is an $18 million dollar business!!!

We are firm at BIRD in our belief that Toxic Marijuana Syndrome is a direct result of ingesting highly toxic chemicals, such as pesticides and insecticides, via the marijuana plant itself and using the one hitters that become very hot, releasing toxins. There are many sources of toxins and we know that the brain has no mechanism to remove these toxins once they enter the brain. These chemicals were never meant to be introduced to the human brain. TMS is real. It must be dealt with and the young people must be treated for it.

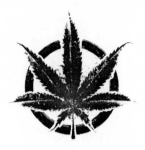

MEDICAL MARIJUANA

California, which was the first state to use weed for medical purposes, developed the California Medical Marijuana Law. This law specifies that in order to get a medical marijuana card for health reasons you must have the following qualifying conditions; Arthritis, Cachexia, Cancer, Chronic pain, HIV or AIDS, Epilepsy, Migraine headaches, Multiple Sclerosis or any debilitating illness deemed appropriate by a licensed Medical Doctor. The state offers phone numbers and a web site to assist and to list doctors who will prescribe medical marijuana. At the time this book was written, there was no possession limits and individuals could cultivate marijuana for their own medical use with the card.

Proposition 215, or the **Compassionate Use Act of 1996** allows patients with a valid doctor's recommendation, and the patients' designated Primary Caregivers, to possess and cultivate marijuana for personal medical use. Since 1996 it has been expanded to protect a growing system of collective and cooperative distribution. The Huffington post posted the following statement on 5/24/14_California is amending its laws and bills are being moved thru the assembly. Although growing and use began in 1996, the state still did not have a set of standards guiding the counties production and sale of the plant. Local government had been in charge.

There have been raids on growers and dispensaries due to the status of THC and its classification. The Obama administration has been less combative in states such as Colorado, which has many more comprehensive regulations, unlike California which will vote again on legalization in 2016, having had it rejected in the first vote. In fact, the state of Colorado was just awarded 12 million dollars for medical marijuana research.

The American Journal of Psychiatry commented on the passage of proposition 215 specifically regarding research on medical marijuana. They stated that The University of California established a Center for Medical Cannabis Research (CMCR) with the central purpose of coordinating rigorous scientific studies to assess the safety and efficacy of cannabis and compounds for treating medical conditions. The funding for CMCR is the result of law SB847 passed by the state legislature and signed into law by Governor Gary Davis. Legislation calls for a three year program overseeing objective high quality research that will enhance understanding of the effects of medical weed.

The following are a few studies being conducted by The CMCR, directed by Igor Grant, M. D.

- One study is looking at sleep and medical marijuana to see if weed is effective in treating pain In HIV and to help assist patients with sleep problems. A Hypothesis is being tested to prove that sleep is enhanced by marijuana.
- Cannabis for treatment of HIV related peripheral nucropatas
- Vaporization as a smokeless cannabis delivery system

- Short term effects of cannabis in its use in therapy with people who have Multiple Sclerosis
- Cannabis in painful Neuropathy
- Effects of cannabis on CD4 immunity in AIDS
- Effects of analgesic cannabis.

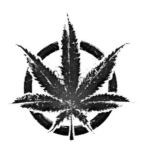

View from the Kids

On a warm fall evening, the youth group meeting that night was exploring the topic presented in a question, "What are you all most passionate about in the world and what do you love the most?" This lively group of young people ages 17-24 dove right into the discussion. Most of the kids shared many of the same passions. Many brought up family and love including self-love and love of good friends. Self-love was a concept introduced many times in group and I could see they were all evolving towards that goal. One young man was very present with his understanding of how Bud had begun to rob him of his passions for both baseball and his ability to receive and give love to his parents. Another 17 year old girl was beginning to understand that she could pursue her passion for creativity in the arts and blessed us with singing a very sweet song. Music has become an essential part of this group and one can break out in a song or rap at any time.

The group was winding down for the night, but they kids were lingering as they will from time to time, not wanting to leave yet. We welcome the ability to move out of rigid clock time. I asked the members if I could ask them something that had been on my mind for a while. I explained that I could use their support in getting some clarity. I was given the green light so I proceeded to ask them to, "Tell me about what you are seeing and feeling about the world you are now growing into?" I wanted to know if they felt they would be supported in fulfilling their passions in life. They were very interested in the question. I asked them if I could jot down what they say and use it in *True Bud* and they said sure.

At this time in this group's development, the members had become very self-motivated, honest and authentic with all things. They shared the following:

1. No one is kind in the world anymore. There would be a much better feeling if we all just started being more kind to each other.

2. Either we are messing the world up or it was handed to us this way by previous generations because there are so many more things to fear now. They also commented on the world's resources and environmental problems.

3. They felt it imperative to find something that would provide enough love to empower them to change things in the world. They felt they needed something good to believe in and work towards and care for. At the current time they just weren't feeling that love.

4. The world has just gotten too focused on the material things and money seems to be the most important thing for many.

5. There is too much technology bombarding us constantly and we don't know how to pull back from it.

6. We have become totally addicted to our cell phones and texting and constantly responding to things without even a chance to think or process stuff. They said they turn off their technology

when they come to group. They welcome that break, but don't know how to pull back from the cells outside of group.

7. We are all over reacting and it's getting worse. Kids are killing other kids in schools. It's crazy that children have guns and can just walk in and alter the lives of some many so drastically. There does not seem to be a stop sign in many heads these days. This stuff is very scary and hard to understand.

8. They expressed that parents are always overreacting too quickly and not really giving them a chance to tell the story or hear their perception of what has occurred. They reported that it is apparent that their parents care and love them, but it often just looks like they are angry. They acknowledged that they cause a lot of reasons for them to react and go off, but feel that their parents are not really listening, just talking at us.

9. The kids had always assumed that Bud was OK and safe to use, but now with all that BIRD is introducing to them they see there may be toxicity. They are beginning to realize that stopping is the way to go but acknowledge that it is hard going thru life feeling everything so intensely

10. There does not seem to be any type of rituals or events that give you a special feeling. Like the Native Americans had that vision quest thing and use peyote buttons, which must have been very deep. They would look for their spirit animal. They wanted to know why they can't do that stuff? They felt it would give them a sense of belonging. I assured them that Bird is not going to be doing the peyote ritual.

11. Everything is moving too fast. They're all driving, walking, doing it all so fast. The tech stuff is also so fast, they never get a chance to stay still. They felt that if they didn't slow down they were going to crash and miss a lot of important things.

12. People are over eating and some don't have enough food. They say there are enough resources around for all of us. They expressed the need to find a better way to help the poor people and others who are less fortunate.

13. The government is in control of everything and also watching everything. There are cameras all over. There are controls, rules, regulations and a lot of taxes. They worry that the government will always know what they are doing and that is not true freedom. They question whether it will get even worse. Even with all this government surveillance and control they can't help prevent all the gun violence in the US.

14. Schools need to be completely redone. There must be better ways to learn and you spend a lot of time there fading out.

At some point they got quiet and had run out of things to say in response to my question. They began to say goodnight. At Bird we have a therapy dog named Shanti They always greet him warmly and say goodnight to him. Some of the kids walk him for me. Shanti is very much loved by these kids. If I miss group and another facilitator does it, they ask if Shanti will still be there working. The dog can tell if a kid has come to group high and he kind of bothers the kid by pulling on his legs and bumping their pockets with his paw. He knows what weed smells like and although I am no expert on pet therapy, I am learning to read him reading the energy of the kids. Many nights I have seen him sit right next to the kid who may be in the most pain or just relapsed. Shanti offers them unconditional love and loves licking and hugging them in his doggy way. I have seen the dog do some things I did not think possible from a dog, like pulling a bag of weed out of a kid's coat. I am pretty sure youth group is Shanti's most favorite thing at Bird.

At the end of group, I grab the dog and head for my car. The kids hangout outside, still not in any rush to leave and enjoying just being with each other. Unlike most other outpatient programs, when it comes to negativity between the kids like smoking weed or buying illegal things from each other, that stuff never goes on at Bird. There is a level of respect for Bird. I have never seen kids support each other in anything but good ways here. I have no reasoning for this at all, but am very grateful this level of trust can exist. It means work will go on and change will happen.

As I drive home, I think about all their comments surrounding their beliefs about the world as it is today. I had deep feelings about what I was hearing. I cannot remember ever having to deal with those things when I was young. I remember the Cuban Missile Crisis and bomb shelters. Yet these kids created some sadness in me that night. I felt we were failing them as adults. I know very few adults who had ever heard kids speak so openly about this kind of stuff. The fears and distrust of the government really surprised me too. I know that something is up if kids are feeling these thigs. I could understand their need to layer up with weed and create some form of insolation between themselves and their world. The Bud serves as a buffer zone, an extra layer of skin protecting them from the insanity. These sensitive kids feel everything intensely and lack the insolation or filters to protect them from such intense emotions.

This fact trumps all other reasons why young people move so deeply into using so much weed. We waste a lot of time on looking at peer pressure, but this is the core issue. We need to help these young people learn how to manage these feelings especially with the supporting brain chemistry they all have. We focus on peer pressure and use it as the main excuse why kids turn to drugs, but it prevents us from looking at the real true core reasons. We are such a drug crazed culture. The kids spoke of rituals, of connecting and belonging. This is something we as adults can provide for them. These kids are left with a longing to know that the future will be there to support them. Bud offers them great insulation and gets them in their comfort zone, where they do not need to feel or dwell on these things.

I am blessed to be a part of these kids' lives. I go home and Shanti is out like a light in two minutes after running around in the meadow discharging all that young energy.

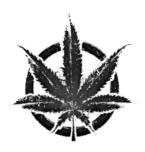

Opening a Dialogue between Parent and Child

There is quite a gap between the inner world of a young person and that of their parents. Any gap in relationship closes communication. As communication shuts down anger, resentment, hurt, and fear arise. When a parent discovers that their child may be using substances they often go to a place of anxiety, fear, and protection. Of course it is all based on love, concern, and the responsibility of being a parent. As a grown person our attitudes and beliefs around a drug like weed are formed. Your stance as the responsible parent is going to be good or bad, right or wrong, yes or no. So many parents have come to us with a bag of paraphernalia they discovered in their child's room. I could open my own head shop with all the pipes, bongs, and other beautifully handcrafted objects used for smoking. A child could have spent $300 on a work of art glass pipe to have it confiscated by their parents never to be returned. Parents are told and will believe that the amazing pipe or one hitter they found are just being held for a close friend. That the bag or bags of weed found are being held for your child's boyfriend because he already got jammed up by his parents.

How about this scenario; A parent comes in to BIRD reporting that their child had a paper bag with $1000 cash, along with tons of dime and twenty weed bags. It is hard to deny what is going on. Right? However I have heard some of the most creative stories and explanations for what was found. Children will bring up the fact that their parents smoked when they were younger, or they still do smoke. They will use this as a defense for their actions. One kid told his folks if they didn't return the bag of cash and weed he would be beat so badly he wouldn't be able to walk!! What's a parent to do? They have illegal drugs in their house. Their child is most likely selling to some of their very own friends' children. What training do any parents have for these scenarios? Does a parent call the police on their own child? Do they throw it all out? Make the child give the money and weed back?

How about the parents who come home from a night out to find twenty very stoned kids and the police waiting for them at their house when they arrive. The police are talking to the parents about obtaining a lawyer, quickly. Not for their kid, but for them! Neglect, reckless endangerment, possession of an illegal substance, and underage drinking. Their child is only 15 and unsupervised. The parent talks to a lawyer and gets scared quickly. They learn they could lose their house and custody of their kid! The lawyer's retainer is coming in at around $3000-$5000. An expensive night out for the parents who were just following their marital therapist's advice to go out alone more and rekindle the relationship. All the neighbors are out on the street, the bright police lights are illuminating them all. Most young people today feel they can do what they want with such a harmless substance like weed. They feel parents will be more understanding since most of them have tried it themselves. They seem to have little understanding of how complicated life can become. Many parents I have spoken with favor legalization for the reasons of making the situations present above a little easier to navigate thru.

All of the above scenarios are constants for many families coming to treatment. Who's fault is it? Is blame and shame the way to go? Surely boundaries have been violated and anger will arise. Often a child may be as angry as their parent and not back down. If any peers are around, they cannot back down. Younger siblings are observing these events and find themselves troubled and fearful for the whole family. The family therapist cannot "fix" these things, not all at once. Yet it is in this rich environment where the work begins. It takes a crisis of some sort for a family to ever get to therapy. The children will often say that the parents are the problem and the parents say it's the kid! "He/She is not like his/her siblings. They don't do these things. There is something wrong with him/her!" After so many years of practice it still troubles me that it takes an event, crisis, problem or legal matter to get families into the office. Knowing things don't feel right in the family and wanting them better is a rare baseline for our institute to see. I often feel that if it were love and concern that brought families in I would rejoice. Pain and suffering seem to be the model we need to create change. I challenge that. It is possible that change could also unfold from love. When the level of love starts breaking down in a family system, all feel it, all know something is wrong. It is just not like it was when love was flowing. Please do not misunderstand. I know love still exists in every family, but it has been replaced by pain and suffering. Communication has broken down. Spending good times with each other becomes less and less frequent. There is more conflict around school, grades, friends, and rules. Being engaged in a constant battle makes it feel like pain and suffering. Blame, shame, and games fly around.

The job of a Family Therapist is to pay attention to "The Life Cycle." Where is this family in the life cycle? Let us take a closer look. The kids are hitting adolescence at the same time that the grandparents are getting older, perhaps sicker and sometimes passing away. The marriage is what it is and one is either happy or silently disappointed in their life partner, maybe no longer even in love and just waiting for the kids to go off to school so they can leave too. Maybe the couple has just gotten stuck and the passion is gone, the sex is rare, they are exhausted from work, life, stress and the new role of caretaking their own parents. Perhaps one of the parents hasn't reached any of their sacred dreams. Maybe they failed, lost their own passion, settled for the job with money and security, but not their true passion. Unspoken of, they can buy toys, have affairs, or get down and fade from view. Their partner misses them but have not a clue where they went or why? It could be the mother took time off from her own career and wanted to be a good stay at home parent. It could be a kid or two already left for school and the house got bigger and emptier and just less joyful. We are very good at staying away from the feelings that all these things create inside us.

Then, on top of all these change of life experiences, you have your 17 year old son smoking weed daily, no longer wanting to hang with you, answering questions with a "later, gotta go." The kid has distanced himself from whatever is going on, yet still feels the pain. Adolescence is a great feeling time in life and a most challenging one too. Brain, hormones, body, and emotional intelligence are all developing. The typical young person doesn't want or seek out their parents' help, insights, or wisdom. Perhaps they feel comfortable reaching out to Grandpa, but things are happening with him and even though you know you are deeply loved, you also know you may lose him soon. They have overheard their parents talking and know something is wrong with their Grandpa, but are not sure what. Young people are so perceptive when they wish to be and when they are not stoned on 80% Dabs. You feel very little on Dabs!

Adolescents have their own questions around who they are and what their world is all about. Struggles with self-image, friendships, worrying about parent's well-being. These are all common place in the adolescent mind. A thought such as, "Is my dad going to have a heart attack, he must have worked 70 hours this week. When did I even see or talk to him last?'" is not uncommon. These so called wild hormones are surging. The child never had acne, but now their face is scaring them and turning off the individuals they desire to be with. Where do they belong? Do they fit in? They realize that weed makes it better! They don't worry as much. Feel as self-conscious. But, their parents are on their case and now drug testing them. Is that even legal? They begin thinking they better go online and get some kind of detox drink or borrow some piss from an old buddy who does not smoke. The Life Cycle! Could there be any other place in time that is as difficult and challenging as this time? There are a lot of questions, uncertainty, and not much communicating. The family therapist has to honor this. Who is the patient here? The family is the patient. Even grandpa, if he is willing.

Thus it is from this place that some connection needs to open up. Some sort of time out from the angry screaming and cursing. Being that this book deals with weed, we know there will be opposing beliefs and opinions. Most times the parent-teen dialogue around weed will be charged. First, we need to remove that charge. The parent can become very skillful around this by pulling back, both emotionally and physically. The parent should be allowed to have their feelings, but need to be encouraged to sit with these feelings and begin to listen deeper to their child. What are their views? Why are they smoking? It may be challenging, but try to let them explain themselves, even if it is not acceptable to you. Practice being present while being with the conflict and the child. Continue to breath. Watch for projection into the future with thoughts of, "Oh my god! She is doing drugs! I knew something was wrong. Is she going to use coke too?" It is important to know that a child will pick up their parents' fears and anxiety and pull back more and may not reveal authentic feelings in fear of having the situation escalate. One need not become a meditation master to be in the here and now in a present way. As a parent use your mind to recall the difficulties and challenges that your own teen years brought you. How intense feelings were at certain times, how fragile you could get, how much work it is for some kids to navigate thru their social world and how that was for you. Slow the process down. If you know you are going to talk at your child, then do not speak, listen, even silence is ok. As a parent you are going to expect that around this subject your child may have a hard time being truthful. They are going to want to protect themselves and friends involved.

I am often amazed witnessing parents blaming their child's friends for their own child's drug use. Parents will quickly start drilling their child about another kid and that group of skateboarders, who they "knew" all along were stoners. I challenge you parents to avoid going there. This is an opportunity for your child to see if they have the ability to take responsibility for themselves. As far as I am concerned peer group pressure is way overrated in our culture as a reason why kids use. I never hear kids talk to me about being or feeling pressured by friends to get high. Yes, a lot of kids want to belong and feel cool, but using is their choice. It is a choice, they are not forced or coerced. Instead, try to gather information from your child. What substances are they using? How long have they been using? How frequently? Do they use alone or with friends? Gather insights instead of looking for someone to blame. Do not position your body opposite your child, but sit beside them, as if you are with them, not against them. A drive in the car is even good. Perhaps even letting them drive so they feel some level of control. Allow them to have their music playing while you talk. Try to enter their world. This will make them feel more comfortable, less on the defensive, and more inclined to open up and trust. Coming at them with everything from your world will not work. Lecturing on how it was when you were their age will not work in that moment. This information may be more useful later in a family therapy session. I find that children are often into hearing about their parents' authentic teen years, but watch the details! They are not as important as your feelings and your own choices.

Here is some advice for the young person, you also need to step back. Your gut reaction will be to defend and lie, but will that truly serve you? Is this new part of your life something that you really understand or know about? How could you? Your brain chemistry is shifting as you grow. Hormones are flowing and smoking weed feels good right now. Can you speak your truth to your parent or parents? Can you believe that no matter how your parents present themselves love is there for you and they are coming from a place of concern and fear? I want you to remember just a year or two back when you were connected to them. Also, I want you to know that substance use is often a brain chemistry event. This brain event is connected to a lot of other events and things in your life. Things that are going to be important for you to know. I want you to think about what your main concern is? Punishment or consequences? Is it anger, judgement or fear around your parents? Are you at a crossroads in your young life where you may need the help and guidance of a parent? Do you feel you need to do and handle everything on your own? Having looked thru some parts of this book, can you be open to what you are reading and know that you are most likely consuming toxins and they are affecting your brain just as it is growing and developing? Finally, are you sure that you know everything and that maybe this would be a good thing to dialogue with a parent or both parents to gain another perspective from those who care? Why limit yourself? It is not about right and wrong. It is about choices and how they affect you. If you are unable, unwilling, or just not sure how to have this dialogue then consult with a good family therapist who understands young people and substance use and the brain. Being willing to seek out help is a powerful intention that never needs to be presented as a consequence or even intervention.

My advice for both parents and children...go into this work with it being for the entire family. All of you need to do some work and need some help. Do not make it just about your child and the weed use.

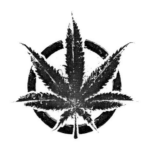

Testing the BIRD Six

I was so impressed with the decision of most of the kids we were testing to stop using Bud and the highly dangerous Dabs, Wax, Butter and Spice. I feel strongly that testing for Nuerotransmitters and metal toxicity and some other excellent tests that affect brain chemistry need to make it into the mainstream Treatment Center around the country. Only a few use Nutrient Therapy and their success rate is higher than ones who do not. Most treatment centers have had a success rate of 20% over the last fifty years. This is not to say inpatient treatment is not needed or that they are not good. The Caron foundation is the one we worked most closely with over the years and they do fantastic work. Especially with young people, where they house and have a separate program that also includes intense family work. Caron is always evolving and adding elements to their program to increase their success rate. They truly care. Even if the centers did not believe in or accept the model of TMS, they have to begin to look at brain chemistry much more closely. It's great that education is big and the group process and spirituality, but if a kid leaves treatment with the same exact brain he walked in with, totally unchanged or understood, the chance of relapse could be much higher.

The concept of brain chemistry testing and looking at the brain and how it is changed thru Nutrients and other interventions is very exciting and adds a major component to treatment that is new and cutting edge. We have never known more about the changes that addiction creates in the receptor sites and brain pathways than at this time.

If a young person leaves treatment with levels of toxicity in the brain and deficient receptor sites, the more susceptible they are to relapse when craving arise. The metal toxicity test revealed that all the chronic weed users had high levels of copper in them. This usually means that their Zinc is also too low and the proper nutrient intervention should be applied. High levels of copper have been connected to lower levels of dopamine and serotonin and higher levels of norepinephrine. This would cause a huge imbalance in the brain and body. It is not uncommon that the features listed below would appear in many individuals with mental disorders if looked at thru the lens of a holistic nutrient therapist practitioner:

A. Excessive Copper, Deficient Zinc
B. Oxidative stress overload
C. Vitamin deficiencies (Specifically vitamin B, C, & D)
D. Lower receptor site activity in some and higher site activity in others

All of these features were observed throughout the testing of the BIRD kids. Of course you can raise the question that perhaps they were not balanced to begin with and that's what moved them to smoke so much. Another hypothesis is that a result of chronic Bud use is the loss of some receptors and the increase of others that should not be too high. The professionals involved in the testing were not able to prove which one was true by our levels of testing, but we will get there. Most kids also were presenting with adrenal fatigue, a rare thing in young people. Adrenal fatigue is something very unexpected in young people, but a major concern to us now and the doctors involved in our testing.

Testing and brain work will raise the success rate significantly if implemented during a long term inpatient stay. Testing and the Nutrients are not that expensive and there are many experts now around the country who could train and set up programs. This could be tied into more research and even better protocols would be developed to send kids home from treatment with the best possible chance at longer term recovery.

I also feel that the chronic weed and dabs users, as well as edible weed addicts would benefit by treatment creating a separate unit just for them. The stories I always get from kids who ended up in rehab just from weed is that they felt very different than narcotic addicts and that the harder addicts often poked fun at the weed kids for even being in a rehab just for bud. A true dope fiend would never go to rehab for bud. They would say it's not even addicting like heroin. At times dope fiends romanticize there use and like to talk a lot about it. Weed is a very different tribal culture, a drug that parents often do with their own kids. The two groups have little in common, other than being addicted to something.

Believe it or not, the chronic weed user's brains take much longer than a heroin addict's brain to return to anything that looks like normal functioning. THC leaves a longer trail than any other drug. It stays in the fat soluble cells in the brain, impacting the firing of neurons. Things like Dabs can be leaving a host of chemicals, from copper to butane in very high levels. While heroin, although a very dangerous illness when addicted, comes in and leaves quick and is often just cut with baby laxative while weed is laced with anything from K2 to PCP to unknown chemicals and synthetic THCs that are still being tried out. These synthetic chemicals will most likely never be tested and if the law is lucky, made illegal the way K2 just was in NYC as a result of volumes of homeless men started showing up in ERs with bizarre symptoms never seen before by any drug.

An ideal substance abuse program would have a unit specifically for Bud users. The Bud kids unit would have more focus on testing, brain repair, and removing the complacency that is growing stronger as it moves towards medical use and legal recreational use. The kids would do indoor rock climbing to raise dopamine and engage in treatment that would target receptor sites. Getting the young people involved in understanding what testing revealed and the power of Nutrient therapy engages them into treatment on a deeper level.

When I sat with a 20 year old whose test showed unusually high levels of mercury, and little dopamine and serotonin receptor activity, the young man was able to understand that his growing brain may not get the chance to grow organically. This seemed to motivate him more than being arrested twice and wrecking two cars, almost losing his life and causing his mother fear, concern and frustration. Until this understanding took place, his view was that bud was safe, non-addicting and totally cool to use. His use of Dabs with the butane tank and copper tubing may have caused the high mercury levels in his brain. We need more testing on young people who use a lot of dabs. It is a new form of using potent THC and, like K2, little is known around what's involved with toxicity and its long term effects. This particular young man was able to shift his beliefs and stop using. He has been doing very well with the brain chemistry repair work that Bird and Systemic Formulas has been trying out on him and others like him. By taking personal responsibility, he changed his life and learned that he is the one responsible for himself, not his mother.

I have seen many young people feel better within a week of being on the right Nutrients. It could be they were born with some genetic depletion and made it worse thru their use. There is a strong link that lower receptor site kids will move towards drugs to raise them and try to feel normal or good. In the beginning they will notice a boost in overall feelings of well-being until further use depletes even more and then depression and anxiety are present in many of the chronic Bud users.

I call upon the medical marijuana industry, now making huge profits and also getting funding for more research to take Birds work to another level and spend more money in educating young people around using weed in excess. We have seen here in this book that medical weed can be organic and do good things for those who are ill. On the contrary, we see weed that is filled with pesticides and toxins.

Edibles will become much more popular for young people as dispensaries open up all over. Just like getting alcohol, kids will find their way to the products made by the medical weed farms. Several kids in our program were already using candies and lollipops and even cooking with high grade oils and butters under such a strong THC influence. Many told us of being able to use while in school because no one is checking the foods they consume for THC. As we stated in the book, edibles grow much stronger as they work their way thru the digestive system greatly impacting the individual's functioning. Being that they take a long time to kick in with the high, young people often smoke too along with eating and are completely baked.

The testing confirms the model we have presented here in True Bud, that young people are developing TMS. The things that these tests revealed supports many of the things that a form of trauma will do to the brain. Young people should not have any methylation issues at all. It is such a critical time in their young brains development. I often can track educational problems to TMS, social problems to TMS, and health related problems to TMS.

R. Wilson also noted that the Bird kids were also significantly high in Cadmium. Cadmium is often high in cigarette smokers, but shows up in excess in Bud users as well. The doctor said that high Cadmium levels in kids so young would have a major impact on their development. This needs to be looked at as a serious concern. A side note to this research is that one kid from the Bird group was so high in mercury that they had never seen anything this high in anyone at 20 years of age. Another young girl from the Bird group was so high in copper that they could not fathom how that could be. She was only 17. The answer to that is in her story in this book. Dabs had a major impact on these two young people's levels.

An interesting note when looking at the nutrient regimen my mother, age 90, was receiving to treat her Alzheimer's disease, we noticed that she was on that same nutrient. Phosophaticyl Serine Powder was included in her treatment along with some other nutrients. In my research with her Nutrient doctor and in my research with bud brain trauma, I found many parallels between the two things. It would seem that the parts of the brain that weed can impact are also impacted in my mother's illness. My mother was the healthiest person I knew. She had been doing and teaching yoga for 60 years and was my very first guru and yoga teacher. She donated all the moneys earned from Yoga to her favorite charities and served many into moving from illness to health. A book like this could never have been written without her insightful teachings. My father and mother just celebrated 70 years together. I'm often reminded of a famous quote from her, "Health is Wealth."

I would recommend a visit to the web site Metabolic Healing.com/ cooper toxicity. It cites the work of Dr. Paul Eck, a well-known copper researcher. On this site, I learned from him that copper sulfate is often sprayed on crops. The doctor also stated that Cadmium from Bud will drive copper back into storage in the body. It will give the young person a good feeling initially, but then cadmium builds up to toxic levels it begins to create problems. You can find an article on springer links, an online site in the review in environmental science and biotechnology, entitled, "Recent findings on the phytoremediation of soils contaminated with environmentally toxic heavy metals and metalloids such as zinc, cadmium, lead and arsenic." (March issue 2004) You can also visit a web site called Rollitup.com and check out information on marijuana plant problems. You will be able to read a guide on Nutrient deficiency and toxicity. You can also read about all the minerals used in the growing process including copper and zinc which both have been addressed in this chapter in regards to testing for toxic levels. On the site springerlink.com there is another article called "Acta Physilogia planiterium" (Sept,2009 Vol 31, issue number 5) which deals with Salicylic acid mediated elevation of cadmium toxicity in hemp plants in relation to cadmium uptake, photosynthesis and antioxidant enzymes. These papers and abstracts are scientific in nature. I don't claim to be a scientist yet I cite them because toxicity in the Bud growing process in plants, soil, nutrients, and insecticides are external epigenetic events contributing to cellular structure and cellular change due to the environment.

I feel we have made a compelling case for Toxic Marijuana Syndrome. I believe that TMS will become better known and more widely understood as a true illness limiting hundreds of thousands of young people's lives at a time when they are just beginning.

(Author's note: We found it very challenging to find a control group of young people who never tried bud. Our intention during testing and now is to still make our T.M.S. project a legitimate scientific research study. We did try with some control groups and we found that there were higher levels of toxicity and receptor site dysfunction. We are going to try to move towards further research and study with more control groups. We are also going to retest our BIRD Six after being on nutrients from systemic formulas. We are hoping more funding becomes available for this important research.)

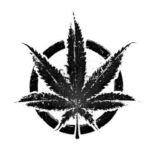

THE EXPERTS' OPINION

Krista Anderson Ross ND, Staff Physician, Labrix Clinical
Services:

Neurotransmitters are viewed as some of the most important signaling molecules produced in the brain, the gut and the adrenal glands.
They communicate information throughout the entire brain and body.
Urinary neurotransmitter testing is currently the Medical Industry's
most reliable and accessible way of measuring both neurotransmitters
in the central nervous system and peripheral nervous system. The production and distribution of neurotransmitters in the central and peripheral nervous systems is influenced by numerous factors: nutritional
status, hormonal imbalances, mental-emotional state, illicit and phar-
maceutic drug use, genetic variances and also routinely used substances
such as caffeine and nicotine.

The laws in the United States in most instances recognize young
people as adults at age 18. However, Experts report that the human
brain doesn't reach maturity until at least age 25. With the recent

legalization of marijuana use throughout many States in the country, the use of marijuana (cannabis), will likely become far more prevalent. And it has already been observed that its use can contribute to neurotransmitter suppression in young people. In fact, Experts in this field (medical marijuana) strongly advise against any recreational use of marijuana before the age of 25, because the brain is still in the process of myelinating (maturation).

The convergence of the laws supporting legal marijuana use in young people in conjunction with unregulated growing and little perviewed commercial paraphernalia industries is also a dangerous combination.

In his book; Scott Gillett has begun to explore the impact of early introduction and repeated use of marijuana on young people and their developing brains, as well as the negative contributory factors of toxic chemicals and heavy metals which are inherent in a majority of marijuana growing and its distribution. And because there is so little scientific research detailing the effects of this drug on young developing brains, we have had to piece together what we know scientifically and find that many important questions remain unanswered:

- Does early marijuana use influence epigenetic variables such as methylation? Or does a genetic methylation variant make one more prone to seek out marijuana?
- Were the low neurotransmitter levels due to preexisting methylation variants and other nutrient deficiencies that predated marijuana use? Or did marijuana use and the additional factors of heavy metals and toxins contribute to the lack of absorption of these nutrients, which then contributed to low neurotransmitter levels? *We know that a methylation variant will contribute to lower than normal monoamine neurotransmitter levels: serotonin, dopamine and norepinephrine, a trend noted in the BIRD*

cases tested through Labrix. As well we know that certain nutrients such as iron, B3, Vitamin C and D and B6 are essential for neurotransmitter production.

- Does preexisting gut dysbiosis predispose one to absorb higher levels of pesticides, toxins and heavy metals associated with marijuana use? Or does the marijuana use and edible ingestion contribute to leaky gut barriers which makes these toxins more readily absorbed?
- Are the nutrient deficiencies associated with marijuana use caused by the leaky gut effect of the toxins associated with its use, or do nutrient deficiencies contribute to a drive to seek out self-medication in the form of marijuana use?
- To what degree do attention deficits play a role in the seeking of marijuana for self-medication?
- To what degree does adrenal insufficiency associated with trauma and stress in a young person's life contribute to seeking out marijuana?

Scientific studies are expensive and finding funding therein can challenging or nearly impossible. Revenues are increasing rapidly in the marijuana industry due to its legalization. Why not mandate some of the revenues for Medical Research? What better way to explore these questions than for research to be funded by the cannabis industry, as well as the pharmaceutical industry which has also jumped on the bandwagon of THC and CBD research and production of medications containing these agents. Thanks to Scott Gillett and his work with the kids at BIRD these questions have been eloquently clarified. Let's put some pressure on the Industry to help answer these questions through solid scientific pursuit. And possibly with better information we can shape and regulate the variables to make marijuana use safer for everyone.

Kathleen Kordas, Holistic Health Practitioner of Nutritional Balancing:

"Kathleen Kordas, Holistic Health Practitioner of Nutritional Balancing, is known for helping others to identify if they are slow or fast oxidizers, have adrenal fatigue, low minerals and metal toxicity. By taking a hair sample and having it analyzed by Analytical Research Labs, the results of these hair analysis testing's (DNA) will help others to discover how balancing their minerals (Calcium, Magnesium, Sodium and Potassium) can rebuild the body and make it healthy.

Scott Gillett, Director of The Briarcliff Manor for Research and Development (BIRD) Institute sent us hair samples of a select group of Marijuana users, and the results showed large amounts of toxicity, such as, Cadmium, Mercury, Copper, Lead and Aluminum. In order to get these toxins out of the body, a Nutritional Balancing Program would be the best direction to take. By following a diet of mostly vegetables and protein, and taking supplements recommended by Dr. Larry Wilson, this will help the Adrenals and Immune System to get stronger and eventually will allow the toxins to leave the body in a non-evasive fashion. If such toxins as Cadmium (from smoking and second hand smoke), Mercury (from silver fillings and fish), Aluminum (from soda cans and deodorants) and bio-unavailable Copper remain in the body, this can and will cause uncomfortable symptoms (Migraines, Depression, Anger, etc.) Along with poor eating habits and metal toxicity, the body can eventually lead to such diseases as Cancer. Yes smoking Marijuana can make us feel great for a time, but there is a consequence that follows the smoking of weed, and that is the buildup of toxins, like Cadmium."

Michael Mendribil, Naturopathic Physician:

"Research by the Briarcliff Institute for Recover and Development has found neurotransmitter imbalances and higher levels of toxic metals in chronic marijuana smokers 16 and 25 years of age. While the absolute source of elevated neurotoxins in the body can not be known, it's likely that toxic marijuana ingestion can play a role.

There are over 400 compounds in marijuana smoke; and depending on methods of cultivation and intake, marijuana may also contain known neurotoxins like cadmium, arsenic, lead and mercury. Once in the body, these neurotoxins contribute to nutrient imbalances and disrupt normal metabolic functions that directly impact brain health and performance, including learning, mood and motivation. Exposure to neurotoxins during the brain's developmental period - up to the mid-twenties according to neuroscientists - can permanently alter the brain's function and structure.

Symptoms of anxiety, depression, fatigue, apathy, anger, and ADHD, among others, are common with excessive use. Sometimes those very symptoms drive individuals to smoke marijuana in the first place. Yet, while smoking marijuana can calm the nervous system and "relieve" symptoms temporarily, it can have unintended consequences and further imbalance the brain and neuroendocrine system.

I believe these symptoms, and those caused by toxic, chronic marijuana use are better treated, in conjunction with behavioral therapy and support, by detoxification and non-toxic nutritional therapies which correct the relative nutritional deficiencies that are often at the root.

While further research needs to be done, it appears that toxins from chronic, toxic marijuana use may play a role in disrupting normal brain function in marijuana addicts."

Ian Jenkins, Systemic Formulas:

"If you are buying your marijuana on the street it is almost impossible to know where it came from and how it was produced. There is no quality control, no industrial standards, no trade certifications that will let you know the quality of what you are getting. You can't even be sure where it came from. Most estimates say that somewhere between thirty and fifty percent come from Mexico or Canada. The other fifty to seventy percent could come from places like Taliban controlled portions of Afghanistan, Columbia, and yes even as far away as china. Grown with water from polluted rivers like the Yangzi River. Water in the Yangzi River is so toxic in some areas that the animals drinking it are dying from toxicity within days. The reality is that we can't know for certain because the majority of import and distribution is still happening illegally. If you are asking yourself why this matters then let me tell you a little about what is happening to the body.

Toxic metals that get into the body from inhalation or ingestion have been found to affect cellular transfer and levels of other important minerals and nutrients that have significant neurological and health effects such as magnesium, lithium, zinc, iron, Vitamins B6 and B12. Based on thousands of hair tests, at least 20% of Americans are deficient in magnesium and lithium, with zinc and iron deficiencies also common. The resulting deficiency of such essential nutrients has been shown to increase toxic metal neurological damage. Cerebrospinal magnesium was found to be significantly lower in both depression and adjustment disorder and in those who have attempted suicide. Studies have also found that heavy metals such as mercury, cadmium, lead, aluminum, and tin affect chemical synaptic transmission in the brain and the peripheral and central nervous system. They also have been found to disrupt brain and cellular calcium levels that significantly affect many body functions, such as cognitive development and degenerative CNS diseases, which results in depressed levels of serotonin, norepinephrine, and acetylcholine; cellular calcium-sodium ATP pump processes affecting cellular nutrition and energy production processes and causing skeletal osteodystery.

In a small pilot study done in New York we found that Late Teen age participants who had smoked marijuana regularly had high levels of toxic heavy metals and impaired neurotransmitter functioning consistent with the larger studies previously mentioned. Interestingly they had a unique underlying thread. Like the larger studies they all had very low production of Serotonin, Dopamine but unlike the larger study they had high levels of GABA and Glutamate. Further study is necessary to draw a definite conclusion but this study suggests that the body is trying to compensate for the impaired dopamine and serotonin channels by increasing GABA and Glutamate production. Very high levels of Glutamate in the brain can have very negative long-term toxicity effects. If we had seen these results from a food that was sold in US stores there would be multi billion-dollar lawsuit and a public uproar over quality control.

The heavy metal toxicity is not the only source of dangerous toxins. For instance, when importers smuggle the cannabis across the border they will do whatever it takes to avoid detection, many shipments are sprayed down with cover up chemicals to throw off the dogs, witch have busted over 20 tons of marijuana in garbage trucks…yep garbage trucks. And what about mold, smoking marijuana with mold can cause serious health problems. Some level of mold is everywhere and normally the body can handle it but in some of the very humid conditions where Marijuana is grown there are often many different species of mold some of which produce chemicals that are deadly in high doses. Without very strict quality control measures mold can and will grow rapidly when shipping any plant and Cannabis is no exception.

About 10% of marijuana on the street came from a garbage truck, over 90% contain some sort of mold, dog hair, pocket lint, high levels of lead and other heavy metals from the contaminate soil where it was grown and the diesel blow off from the vehicles. The chemicals used to keep the bugs and dogs away contain high levels of glyphosate that destroys your internal microbiome. The cover up sprays used to mask the odor during the smuggling process contains chemicals with known irritant and neurotoxic properties.

With all of the combined toxic influences it is not a surprise that we are seeing this kind of physiological reaction and the addictive be-havior. Low Serotonin and Dopamine caused by toxins in or on the Bud are creating a deficit of the feel good neurotransmitters, which in turns creates a craving for marijuana just to feel normal. When they smoke or ingest the cannabis they are adding to the toxic insult and furthering the vicious cycle. More bud = more toxins = impaired neu-rotransmitter function = more cravings = more bud...

At the time of this publication we are In the middle of an adaptive Study using methyl donor supplementation form MORS, and cogni-tive support supplements from Systemic Formulas to stave off the mild cognitive decline associated with this type of behavior and break the ad-diction cycle. Preliminary results are very encouraging but further study is still needed. According to Dr. Morris PHD the body becomes methyl depleted when attempting to detox heavy metals and chemical insults."

1. Assessment, Cincinnati, Ohio webpage EPA spokesman, US. News & World Report, "Kids at Risk", 6-19-2000; & U.S. EPA, Region I, 2001, www.epa.gov/region01/children/outdoors.html
2. Agency for Toxic Substances and Disease Registry, U.S. Public Health Service. Toxicological Profile for Mercury. March 1999.

and Media Advisory, New MRLs for toxic substances, MRL: elemental mercury vapor/ inhalation/chronic & MRL: methyl mercury/oral/acute. Jan 2003. www.atsdr.cdc.gov/mrls.html

3. Lewis M, Worobey J, Ramsay DS, McCormack MK. Prenatal exposure to heavy metals: effect on childhood cognitive skills and health status. *Pediatrics* **89(6 Pt 1):**1010-15. 1992.

4. Anderson RC, Anderson JH. Toxic effects of air freshener emissions. Arch Environ Health. 1997 Nov-Dec;52(6):433–441.

5. Gettman, Jon. "The Supply of Marijuana to the United States." *The Supply of Marijuana to the United States.* Drug Science Org, 2007. Web. 05 Nov. 2015.

6. "Where Does Your Weed Come From?" *Medical Marijuana Advisor.* Medical Marijuana Advisor, 2009. Web. 5 Nov. 2015.

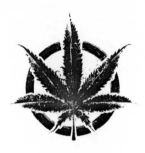

Nutrient Therapy for the Weed Addicted Brain A Guide for Parents

Weed is an addictive substance. I am not going to spend time on the credibility of this. All drugs have the potential to be addictive based on use and lack of control. Much has been learned about weed addiction over the years from young people who are very trusting. WE DO NOT JUDGE. My goal is to keep the dialogue open, to keep people talking. The position of this book is to be an ally to young people; an informative ally. Once you are trusted, the truth reveals itself. At times this book will use tools like questionnaires to evaluate a young person's circumstance but the buck stops there. We do not criticize. Whatever the circumstance, anyone reading this already senses or knows weed as an addictive substance. They also often have no idea where they fall on the spectrum. Are you a habitual smoker, a casual smoker, or a social smoker? The spectrum looks like this;

1. Random Smoker: experimenting, smokes just a few times

2. Weekend Warrior Smoker: smokes at parties, parks, occasionally at home, and in social situations.

3. Rain or Shine Smoker: four times a week regardless of the day or time of day, rain or shine. You primarily smoke to get thru stuff that is boring or to chill out from stress.

4. The Grind Smoker: Daily smoking, after school or work, in the evening to help with sleep and to get thru responsibilities.

5. Chimney Smoker: smoking more than once a day. You are occasionally waking and baking to smoke before school or work. You look forward to smoking, thinking about smoking, and devote energy to use.

6. Cheech and Chong or Chronic Smoker: smoke several times daily, alone at times. You hoard your stash. Sometimes you conceal your use. You may have money problems due to use. Relationships shifts based on use. Going to work or school is not a priority. Using weed to get through life and the inability to stop even when you want defines the Cheech and Chong Smoker. The loss of choice coupled with a loss of appetite, mental confusion, respiratory issues could mean you are using laced weed.

High functioning weed users may be so dependent that they need to smoke a lot just to get a buzz. However these people function fine because their brain chemistry has compensated due to extreme use. Loss of Gaba in the brain prohibits feeling the calming, mellow effect of weed. There is not a lot of motivation for these kids but they are still able to get through events like school, work, and family gatherings.

The challenge here is to pinpoint a person's needs and develop a treatment plan to mirror their needs. All young people are present on the spectrum above. They need to be looked at as individuals and not lumped together as being the same. Treating them with dignity and respect is the key. Being open to their process and understanding is how you gain that trust. They need to see that you know your stuff. They need to be engaged. They need to feel at home in the setting where the "change" will happen and have a voice in that change. Of course the most important ingredient is love. They need to be loved and told so in a way that is authentic and real. Give time to that and let it come to you. Let it reveal itself. Breathe. Hang with them. Don't push the understanding of their stress or challenges in life. Breathe and let it release from them.

You also would be wise as parents and/or family members to understand your family dynamic and where your young person fits in that. This is not just about your social relations to them. Genetics and illnesses, epigenetic are meaningful chapters in this story of "change". Every family has a story and you need to know it. Be patient with those you work with and at times you have to think like a detective to get that full story. The people who have had enough of their weed use and want to quit have an options. Nutrient Therapy along with a regular traditional treatment plan can make a difference. However remember the key ingredient is love and understanding.

BIRDS Nutrient Profile for BUD

A Nutrient Shake is essential with all the needed ingredients. Here are some options:

1. Spirutien, Spirulina shake in many flavors made by Natures Plus
2. True Hope EMPR Power Shake – www. Truehope.com
3. Three Shake options from Systemicformulas.com – all excellent products.

We would recommend you blend the shake with coconut water or milk, almond milk, rice milk, fruit (if your diet allows), ice or juices. Take in AM with your Nutrients to start your day.

Supplements:

- Zinc – 25-50 mg daily for first month to build lost zinc back up.
- Omega 3 fatty acids – 3000 mg daily or Lovaza (a script from your doctor is needed for this, but works very well with our plan).
- GABA – 3,000 mg for first three months at night or can use sublingual GABA calm by Natures Plus as needed during your day, around five-ten times a day. You cannot overdose on GABA.
- NC Calm and Relaxa from Systemic Formulas – 2-4 capsules every four hours
- CoQ-10 – 100 mg daily
- Vit C – 2,000 mg daily
- L-Lysine – 1500 mg daily
- Tyrosine – 1500 mg daily
- DLPA-Phentlanine – 500 mg daily
- Headaches during early withdrawal – Magnesuim and Calcium – 300 mg of each

Brain Chemistry repair and food:

- Restore by Systemic Formulas
- Neurosyn by Systemic Formulas
- 5HTP – 100 mg daily
- Same E – dose on bottle or packet

- Cognizin – GPC choline and Citicholine – dose on bottle
- Alpha GPC – 400 mg daily
- Phosphaticyl Serine Powder - dose on bottle
- California poppy (dose on bottle) used with GABA to reduce cravings. Take at night, may be sedating, but also okay in first two weeks of withdrawal.
- Brain Recovery – AM-PM-Cell support Plus – Sold on Dr. Cass' website – www.cassmd.com/products.
- The Pro Recovery Diet by Patrice Reiss (director of A.A.S.)
- Julia Ross author of The Mood Cure and several excellent CD's on pot.

The plan to use these nutrients involves a very lengthy evaluation at the Institute. The items that we feel are needed will be checked and those are the ones you buy and obtain. It is not necessary to take everything on the above list. Each client is different and testing is sometimes part of the evaluation for toxins and receptor site activity, this evaluation is made specifically for young people. The parent will be involved as well as pediatricians and psychiatrist if appropriate. A full medical history is required including medications being taken and any other substances, including Alcohol, which you also may have used or abused. This Nutrient plan is truly useless unless you are ready, willing and going to stop Bud now! We understand that will be difficult and we are here to assist and support you. Some more things that will assist you are: steam baths and saunas, a lot of drinking water and fresh juice, going to 12 step meetings such as AA, NA and MA, indoor or outdoor rock climbing and other forms of exercise.

This nutrient plan is also a great plan to help with post-acute and regular withdrawal. It is a great way to navigate through recovery with brain, body, and spirit. Here is a Nutrient plan specifically to help with withdrawal and to stay weed free. It is important to note that it will not be effective if weed is still used. Complete abstinence is required:

1. Zinc-2-0mg daily for first month.
2. Omega 3 fatty acids-3000mg daily
3. Gaba-3,000mg daily in the evening
4. NC Calm and Relaxa from Systemic Formulas - 2-4 capsules every four to six hours.
5. CoQ10-50-100 mg daily
6. Vitamin C-2,000mg daily
7. L-Lysine-1500 mg daily & Tyrosine-same mg
8. DLPH-Phenylnine-1500mg daily
9. Magnesium and Calcium-300mg daily. Primarily for headaches and apathy.-

To deal with the lack of energy, low motivation, and loss of apatite:

a. Walk
b. Drink a lot of water
c. Eat a diet high protein
d. Avoid sugar and avoid stimulants like red bull, coffee, and energy drinks with natural stimulants.
e. Exercise (for example Yoga or Tai-Chi)
f. Withdrawal is a reality and so is Post-Acute Withdrawal. So there is no shame in going to AA or NA if you feel the need or your loved one needs.
g. Indoor and outdoor rock climbing will help to raise the receptor sites dopamine and endorphins and impact the brain and body in a positive way.

When speaking of Post-Acute Withdrawal Symptoms (PAWS), keep in mind that certain withdrawal symptoms may linger much longer with weed than with other substances. THC stays in the body for quite some time. It is not uncommon to have someone test positive for THC six weeks after stopping use. The most common symptoms for recovering smokers are; headaches, apathy, loss of appetite, mental confusion, feelings of anxiety or panic, insomnia, and anger.

The Nutrient Protocol needs to be supervised by a health professional coupled with a complete evaluation and medical exam. Using Nutrient Therapy for addictions and mental health is becoming more mainstream in our culture as we learn more about the ways nutrients impact upon the brain. A great reference for this is The Alliance for Addiction Solutions. Young people are going to need help. Getting consistent nutrients into their system daily is that help. It is advised to consume the above nutrients with some type of protein shake at the start of the day. It's all about finding a system that works for the brain to recover and heal.

CPSIA information can be obtained
at www.ICGtesting.com
Printed in the USA
LVOW08s0814100217

523826LV00001B/77/P